GET

the

GLOW

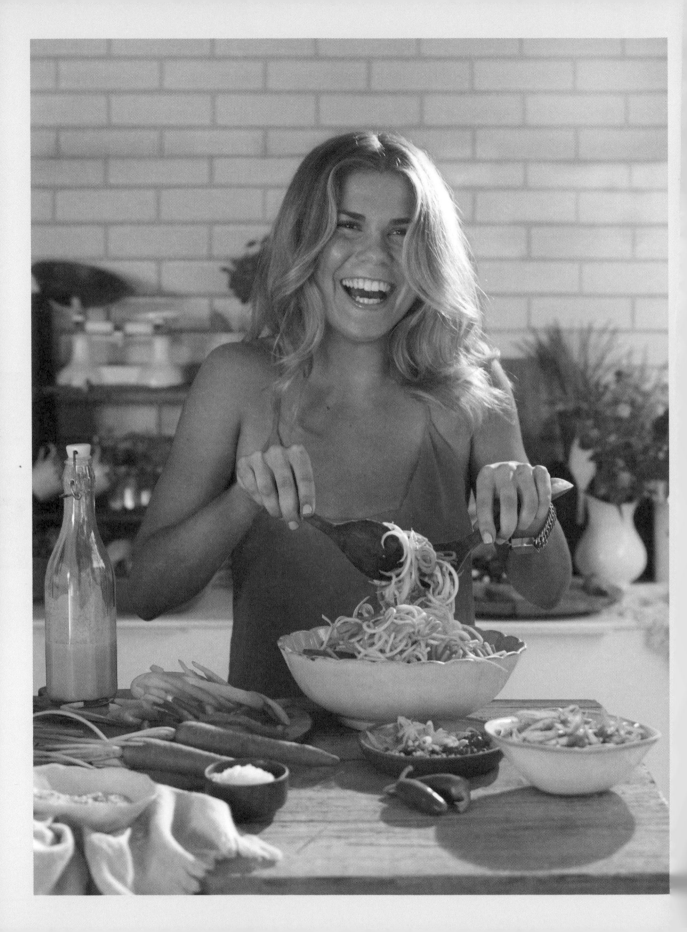

GET
the
GLOW

100 delicious and easy recipes that will
nourish you from the inside out

MADELEINE SHAW

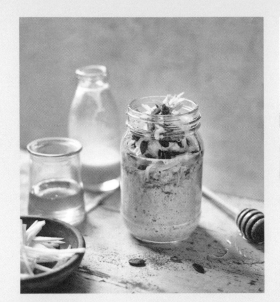

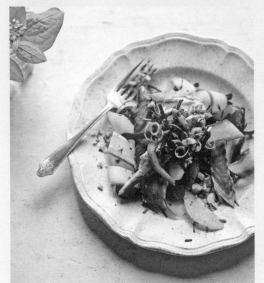

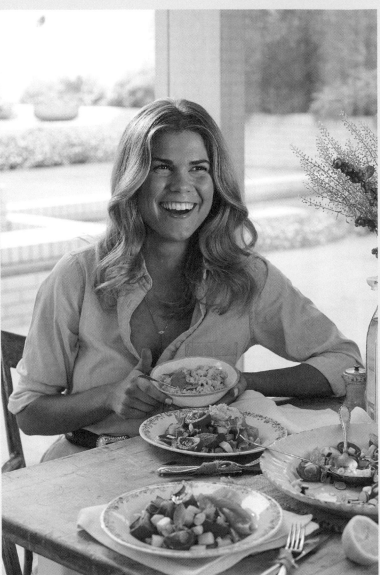

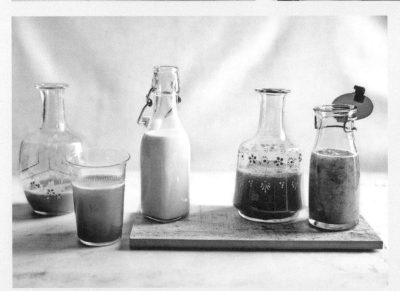

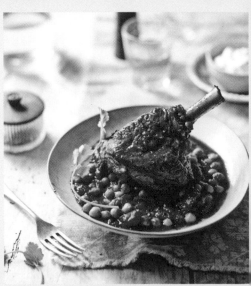

contents

introduction

This book was written for you. It brings together all the food I love, along with all of the lessons I have learnt and the experiences I have been so blessed to enjoy. Most important of all, it is here to enliven the hottest, happiest and healthiest you, so you can shine from head to toe and really get the glow!

my story

Not so long ago I used to wake up foggy-headed every morning, dragging a second day hangover. I would pinch my flabby stomach, stare into my lifeless eyes and groan in despair. I suffered from terrible IBS, my belly was bloated, I felt tired and uncomfortable. My skin was dull, my hair lifeless and my head quite lost.

How on earth had I got to this place?

The world seemed hard to control, so I decided to control the only thing I felt I had the power to…food.

I realised that controlling this aspect of my life allowed me to block out the other uncontrollable things. It started to consume me; I thought about food 24-7. I counted calories all day. I felt nervous in social situations around food and never ate anything that could potentially fatten me up. I felt faint and never quite there. I would binge and then experience horrendous 'come-downs', beating myself up for failing to stick to 'the plan'.

Being thinner and having 'control' over my life was supposed to make me happier…but it really didn't. But upon leaving school I embarked on a journey.

Since the age of seven I had been obsessed with Australians (which might have had something to do with *Crocodile Dundee*!). So, on hitting 18, I made it my mission to spend time in this paradise.

From the minute I landed in Oz I felt at home. It was the strangest feeling. A sense of calm washed over me and I knew deep in my gut that I had to live there – that somehow this place would help me uncover the true me.

Being a tad impulsive by nature, I applied to Sydney University and was accepted a few weeks later, so I returned to my London home, got my gear and hopped on a plane to Oz.

It was a bold move and so many people thought I was mad. I was, of course, very far away from home. However, as I sat on that 22-hour flight, I repeated, again and again under my breath, a line from *The Alchemist*, by Paulo Coelho:

'Remember that wherever your heart is, there you will find your treasure.'

This was totally true for me.

I was blessed to find a job working in an organic café in Bondi. I blossomed there. It was quite amazing; I had never experienced a job that didn't feel like a job. It was so effortless. It sounds corny but it felt like an expression of who I was. I learnt so much about the importance of food to our health, mood and general well-being. I realised that my body had been starved of proper whole foods, nourishment and love. The café was filled with the most miraculous people I had ever met; people who taught me how to properly prepare, source and cook food.

Moving to Sydney was the wake-up call I needed. It made me really want to take care of my body. I felt inspired to jump out of bed, to catch the sunrise or paddleboard the shores. Eating a wholesome diet enabled me to experience life on another level. My IBS cleared and for the first time I felt well. I studied nutrition, created my blog and moved back to London to spread the message of healthy eating.

I began teaching my Get the Glow programme in 2012 with the aim of helping others overhaul their health through food, and I've since helped countless men and women to ditch the fad diets and make healthy eating a way of life.

I genuinely feel like a changed woman because of the education I had in Oz, and this is why I feel so passionate about sharing my knowledge with you. With this book, over the course of six weeks, you'll learn how to nourish your beautiful body so you can get not only an outer glow but an inner one too.

These are my top tips to help you get through the next 6 weeks:

- **Prepare:** Decide how many recipes you're going to cook and do your shopping and prepping for the week on a Sunday.
- **Buddy-up:** Studies show you are more likely to start and succeed at a new diet or lifestyle if you're doing it with somebody else.
- **Be your biggest cheerleader:** Write down little reminders and encouraging words to give you the motivation to keep going (follow me on Instagram @madeleine_shaw_ for daily inspirational quotes).
- **Put it out there:** Tweet it, Facebook it and tell it to all your friends. You will be more inclined to stick at it if you have the world watching.
- **Manage your mindset:** Don't despair and fixate on what you have to give up; instead focus on all the exciting new foods you will be filling your plate with. It's going to be a tasty affair, I promise.

I hope you enjoy this book and that by the end you'll believe that healthy eating should be a way of living, not just a monthly 'fad' or 'phase'. I would love more than anything for this book to help inspire you to fall back in love with life and yourself.

Madeleine

six week programme

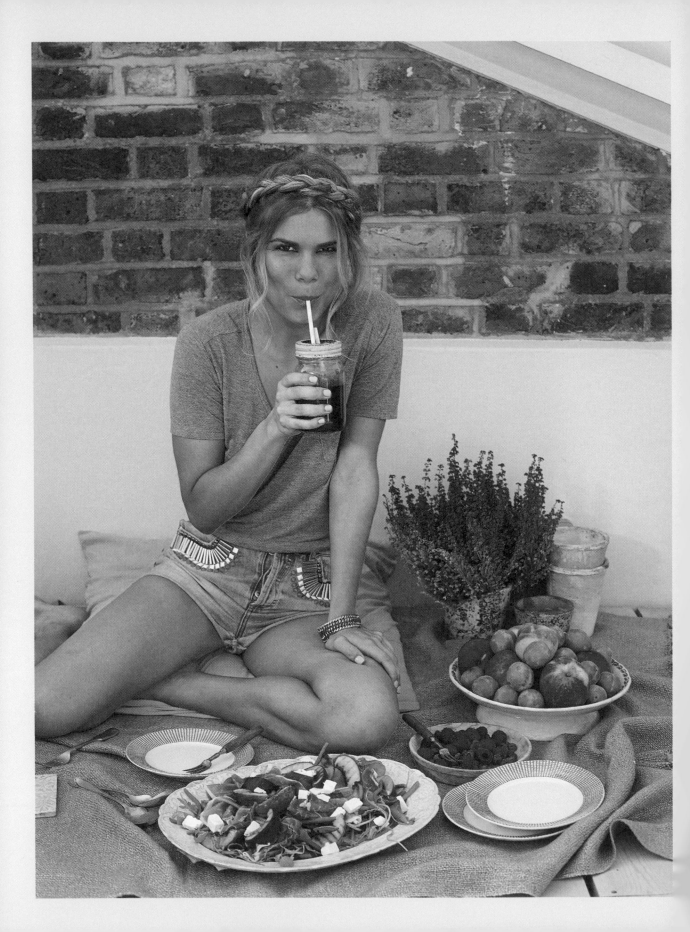

Our skin is a reflection of our inner health. This week we are ditching the junk to get the outer glow.

you are what you eat

Do you feel foggy-headed? Have tired, dull skin, and most of the time (let's be honest)...feel like crap? Can you really eat only one biscuit and walk away?

If the answer to any of these questions is 'yes' – well, I think it's time to kick that sugar monster.

desert the sugar

'Everything in moderation.' Right? 'A little bit here and there won't hurt . . .'

These are our justifications when it comes to sugar. However, it isn't always as simple as that.

Historically sugar was an expensive rarity, but as trade with sugar-producing countries increased, it has become cheaper and cheaper, and we are now eating more sugar than ever before.

The average person in Britain consumes about 700g of sugar per week – that's 140 teaspoons! So what is this sugar doing to our bodies, and why do we need to quit?

- **It sends us out of whack:** High sugar intake upsets important hormones in our bodies – especially insulin, the energy-storage hormone.
- **It can make us fat:** When our blood sugar levels are high we use a certain amount for ready energy, but the rest we store as fat.
- **It masks the taste of other food:** Sugar trumps all other tastes; it dulls them so you will think you only enjoy the sweet stuff. When you come off it, you will actually be able to taste food properly again!
- **Sugar affects your mineral and nutrient absorption:** It also contributes to bloating and indigestion.
- **It's pointless:** Most sugary foods lack

needed nutrients, so in effect you are eating 'empty' calories.

- **It's bad for you:** Studies on people around the world show that sugar in the diet may be linked to a range of metabolic problems including obesity, diabetes and cancer.

sciency stuff simplified

The rate that sugars in food are broken down and absorbed into the bloodstream is called the food's glycemic index (GI).

Sugars from low-GI foods are absorbed slowly, leading to a gradual rise in blood sugar levels. However, sugars from high-GI foods are absorbed more quickly, causing a rapid rise in blood sugar levels.

As sugars move into the bloodstream, they trigger the release of insulin from the pancreas. Insulin acts to remove sugars from the bloodstream for storage in our cells.

The other hormone involved in our energy balance is leptin. This hormone signals to your brain how much energy is available in your body and what to do with it.

A substance called dopamine, produced in the reward centre of our brains (a collection of brain structures that regulates anything pleasurable) controls our overall energy balance. It gives us that sense of satisfaction and reward when we eat. In contrast, the 'fullness' hormone leptin normally keeps this in check by suppressing the effect of dopamine – so we ease off eating.

When our energy levels (intake and output) are in balance, we burn energy at a normal rate, and feel really good.

But a sudden hit of sugar requires a rapid release of insulin to match it, and we get an insulin 'spike'. A spike in our insulin levels can block the way leptin normally signals fullness to the reward centre in our brains. This blocking effect simply primes our appetite for more sugar.

Continuing to eat sugary foods can increase our tolerance to the way they affect our reward centre to such an extent that we find it hard to resist scrounging for more. So sugar effectively creates an appetite for itself . . . and the addiction begins.

hidden sugars

The big problem with refined sugar is that it is EVERYWHERE. Not just in ice cream, biscuits and cupcakes.

Among the worst offenders are the hidden sugars that are found lurking in so-called 'healthy foods', where sugar may be added to mask the lack of flavour in low-fat products. You think you are being good when you choose these, but in reality they can make you more inclined to binge later. Hidden sugars are found in:

- soft drinks, especially sports drinks (just 500ml of many popular fizzy drinks contains the equivalent of 17 cubes of sugar)
- low-fat and diet products
- most breads and bread products (rye and sourdough are low sugar and my Quinoa Bread, see page 96, is sugar free)
- most commercial soups
- almost all processed foods
- many breakfast cereals (swap for my Raw Berry Buckwheat Porridge or Simple Overnight Bircher, pages 80 and 70)
- condiments such as mustard, BBQ sauce, ketchup and chilli jam.

what about fruit?

It's true that fruit contains sugar. However this sugar is metabolised very differently from white table sugar. Fruits contain fibre (which slows down the digestion of the sugar), phytonutrients (which improve metabolic function) and heaps of vitamins (these fill you up, so you don't consume as much). Aim to eat no more than one to two portions of fruit a day, and stick to low-sugar fruits such as berries, kiwi, grapefruit and green apples. High-sugar fruits, such as mango, pineapple, bananas and dried fruit can be consumed a few times per week.

what benefits will i see?

So now you know why you should ditch the junk and where it lurks, it's time to find out about all the lovely rewards you will reap.

- **Your skin will glow:** Sugar reacts with proteins in our bodies, causing them to form advanced glycation end-products, which age the skin. Sugar causes a breakdown of collagen in the skin, so when you quit the sweet stuff your skin will become radiant and resilient.
- **Your food addiction will diminish:** Obsessing about food all day long? Sugar makes you hungry all the time. Say goodbye to this once you quit.
- **Weight will fall off:** You'll lose pounds and you'll be proud of your leaner, healthier physique.
- **You will feel happier:** When you quit sugar your energy becomes more stable, and so does your mood. Time and time again clients tell me they feel less anxious/irritated/grumpy.
- **You will learn to love your kitchen:** Quitting sugar means no more processed foods, which means more home-cooked meals from scratch! This is an easy way to make your plate more nutritious and delicious.

the break-up

One of the things that makes quitting sugar so hard is our emotional relationship with it. On the whole, when things go wrong we turn to the sweet stuff, and – hey presto – when birthdays and other celebrations come around, there's cake again too.

The easiest way to get over this is to replace sugar as a reward with something else: like one of my Raw Superfood Balls (see page 102), a herbal tea, paint your nails, go for a walk or treat yourself to a little pampering!

I promise you – once you get off the sweet stuff, it's amazing how little you will crave it.

I'm not saying this is going to be easy and, yes, you can get withdrawal symptoms. These may show up as headaches, the grumps, irritability or energy slumps.

But push through! When you emerge on the other side you will be greeted with boundless energy, glowing skin and big smiles all round.

take action now

This week is all about making simple changes to your diet by quitting all added sugar. Remember, that's no:

- white sugar, brown sugar or cane sugar
- sugary drinks like canned fizzy drinks, tonic water, fruit juices, squash, etc. Swap for sparkling water and a slice of lime or lemon, coconut water or herbal tea
- cakes, biscuits, ice cream or sugary treats. Keep healthy snacks on hand: a handful of nuts, a pot of natural yoghurt, a boiled egg, a slice of smoked salmon or some fresh berries
- processed foods with sugar in the ingredients
- diet/low-fat foods
- jams and sweet spreads. Use avocado or a soft-boiled egg instead

I do hate the word 'no', and I am sorry for saying it so many times, but you have to be strict with yourself to get the most out of this experience.

sweeter alternatives?

OK, so we've learned that the sweet stuff isn't doing us any favours. But what if, like me, you love the taste of something sweet? Thankfully, there are healthier ways to satisfy your sweet tooth. Here are the sugars to miss and the ones to enjoy. It's simple: just switch bad for good.

Sugars to avoid:

- **Agave**: This is the new 'healthy' sugar everyone is pouring into their green smoothies. However, on the whole it is highly processed and contains 80% fructose sugar. Most agave doesn't resemble the original agave plant in the slightest (switch this one for honey).

- **High-fructose corn syrup:** The nastiest of them all, this one is super-processed and can be highly addictive (switch for coconut sugar).
- **Aspartame:** Found in diet drinks, sweets and chewing gum; this stuff could be toxic and is something you need to ditch (switch for stevia).
- Others to watch out for: **sweeteners, dextrose, glycerol, fruit juice concentrate, sorbitol, sucanet, grape syrup** and, of course, **standard table sugar.**

Better substitutes:

- **Honey:** A great sweetener that you will see in many of my healthy desserts. Bursting-full of antioxidants, vitamins and minerals, this delight also has healing properties for the digestive tract. Aim to buy quality raw or manuka honey where you can.
- **Stevia:** This is a super-sweet herb that originates from the South American stevia plant. It is tremendously sweet (300 times sweeter than sugar), so don't start putting whole cubes of it in your cuppa.
- **Coconut sugar:** This is a simple substitute for sugar in cake recipes. It doesn't actually taste of coconut (in fact, it has more of a caramel taste). It is a very sustainable sugar and abundant in vitamin C and amino acids.
- **Dates:** Loaded with fibre and B vitamins, they also act as a great binder in many of my raw desserts.
- Others to use in moderation: **xylitol, brown rice syrup, maple syrup.**

Although these are healthier sugars, try and go easy on them. You want your palate to adapt to less sweetness, and you'll find it easier to make the transition if you use the alternatives sparingly. Let's aim for once or twice a week.

top tips to make sugar-free easy:

- Try to start from scratch by making your meals at home.
- Clean out your cupboards, read the food labels, and throw out anything that contains added sugar. With these out of the house you are less likely to cave in at a weak moment.
- Start moving that booty! Exercise is a great helper – it takes your mind off food.
- Try liquorice and peppermint tea (it tastes super-sweet and aids digestion).

- Try adding some cinnamon to your breakfast – this can help stabilise your blood sugar levels and make the rollercoaster journey a little smoother.
- Start every day with warm water and lemon – this is really cleansing for the system, it helps rehydrate the cells and get the digestive juices fired up ready for a sugar-free brekkie.
- Up your protein intake – this really helps sugar cravings. Good sources of protein are fish, grass-fed meat, free-range eggs, nuts, seeds and quinoa.
- Think positive. You can do this! (More about this in Week 3.)

Now you're prepped, ready to take charge of your food and all set to embark on a junk-free diet. To help you through this stage, I've compiled a list of questions that might pop up along the way.

Q&A

Q: What happens if I slip up?
A: Don't beat yourself up! One treat won't hurt you, but don't make it into a bad week. The best thing is to start afresh with the next meal.

Q: I'm getting the worst headaches, help me!
A: Coming off sugar can be like a savage hangover if you're used to having a lot of it. The body is detoxing, and it takes a couple of days to a week to get your system feeling normal. Drink lots of water to get through it. I like to mix 2 teaspoons cider vinegar with warm water; it may be an old wives' tale, but it works. Remember, it takes time to repair the damage, and this isn't a race to the finish line. I'm building you with bricks, not sticks.

Q: My usual morning cereal has sugar in it. What are some break-fast alternatives?
A: Sugar lurks in most breakfast delights. Opt for plain oats, and add yoghurt, cinnamon and nuts to liven it up. Go for rye bread or my Quinoa Bread (see page 96) with nut butter, smoked salmon or eggs on top.

Or make a quick breakfast bowl with natural yoghurt, seeds, berries and toasted coconut flakes. I have so many easy and scrumptious breakfast recipes in the recipe section that you can start munching on now.

Q: *What about alcohol?*

A: Binge drinking definitely causes that belly bulge. When we drink excessively our body becomes toxic, our liver works harder to reduce the toxicity and weight piles on easily. Excessive alcohol makes our skin dry and our mood dreadful … at least the next day. Another issue with alcohol is that it makes us eat terribly; it throws the regime out the window and makes you crave like crazy.

I'd aim to give it up for the whole 6 weeks to give your body a break. However, if that's not an option, stick to the 'cleanest' drinks such as red wine, tequila or spirits with soda water as your mixer. Aim to consume only three drinks per week, and sip them slowly. Avoid the following like the plague: cocktails, beer, tonic water (very sugary), and any spirit mixed with a fizzy drink (including so-called 'diet' or 'no sugar' fizzy drinks).

In social situations I find if you always have a drink in your hand – like a sparkling water and lime – people leave you alone; it passes off as something alcoholic and you don't get pestered. If you're empty-handed it's pretty much guaranteed you will be bullied to the bar.

Q: *What do I do if I'm hungover?*

A: I know, I know, alcohol is part of our culture nowadays – so if you're going to have a proper session, it's good to recover the healthy way.

- **Step 1:** Rehydrate – drink at least 3 litres of water that day, and add a pinch of sea salt to help restore lost minerals.
- **Step 2:** Get some electrolytes back into your system with a bottle of coconut water and a banana.
- **Step 3:** Eat some veggies. Your body needs a variety of nutrients to heal the damage. Stay away from the kebab store and instead make my Fried Eggs with Bacon and Roast Vine Tomatoes or Breakfast Smoothie Bowl (pages 90 and 98).
- **Step 4:** Sleep it off. Don't try and sweat it out at the gym; take the day to relax.

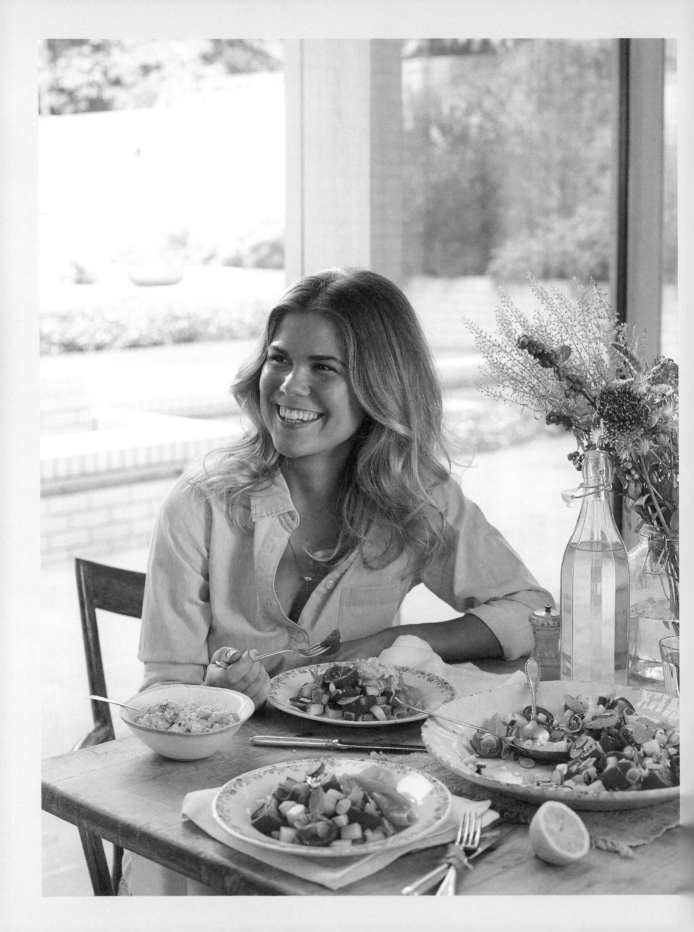

FAT:

friend

OR FOE?

week two

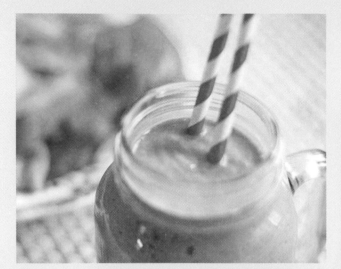

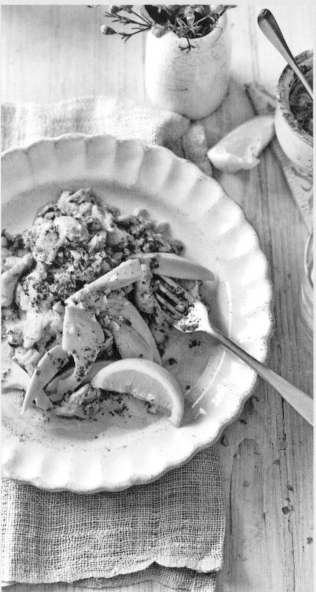

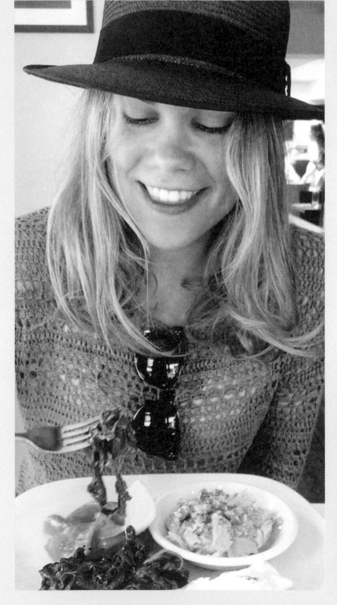

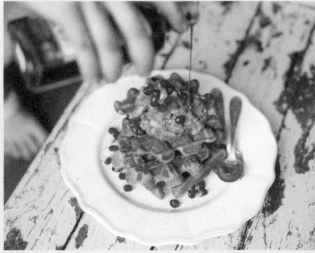

So you've ditched the sugar, now it's time to get the foodie glow.

escape the low-fat mind-trap

It's time to switch your low-fat habits for a love of healthy fats. Now, before you run a million miles with your full-fat phobia, hear me out . . .

I know past diets have told you that if you eat fat you'll gain fat. But, low fat = high sugar. When food manufacturers extract fat, they pack in the sugar to mask the lack of flavour. The high sugar content in these so-called healthy alternatives make you eat more and buy more (clever marketing, hey?). When I tell my clients to eat whole (full-fat) yoghurt they look at me in shock. You're probably thinking exactly the same thing . . . *isn't it going to make me fat?*

It's actually the opposite. Full-fat tastes better, it fills you up so you don't eat as much, it nourishes your beautiful body, and it will help curb those sugar cravings. 'Full-fat' isn't even loaded with fat – it's just how it was naturally designed to be.

Swap this:	For this:
Diet salad dressings	Olive oil and vinegar
Low-fat yoghurt/ crème fraîche/sour cream	Full-fat/natural/ Greek yoghurt/ crème fraîche/sour cream
Low-fat cheese	Full-fat/normal cheese
Diet bars or snacks	My Raw Superfood Balls (see page 102)

why is fat so good for us?

- Healthy fats provide essential fatty acids that your body physically can't produce for itself.
- Healthy fats are concentrated sources of energy.
- They help to maintain your cell membranes.
- They keep the nervous system in working order.
- They boost the body's immune system.

- They help you have healthy hormones.
- They act as carriers to enable the body to absorb super-important fat-soluble vitamins A, D, E and K.
- They also slow down absorption, so our feeling of fullness and satisfaction after a meal lasts longer.
- They also make your food taste delicious!

what healthy fats should i eat?

Healthy fats are a crucial part of a well-balanced meal, so aim to get them in every meal. Here is a list of great sources of healthy fats:

- **Coconut oil:** Packed with medium-chain triglycerides that get used upfront as energy. It's the best oil to cook with, as it has a high smoking point and doesn't denature with heat.
- **Olive oil:** Bursting with antioxidants that help prevent cell degeneration in your skin, and counter ageing. Perfect for drizzling over salads and roasted veggies.
- **Avocado:** Packing an impressive load of goodness, avocados are a great source of biotin, which helps to prevent dry skin, brittle hair and nails. Throw it into salads and smoothies or have with eggs in the morning.

- **Nuts:** Loaded with the amazing antioxidant vitamin E that helps to keep your face looking rejuvenated and youthful. Enjoy a handful as a snack, or add to smoothies and salads.
- **Seeds:** High in zinc, which helps maintain collagen and promotes new skin growth. Toast them in coconut oil and cinnamon and toss over your breakfast bowl.
- **Pasture-raised meat:** Rich in omega-3 fatty acids that reduces inflammation and redness in the skin.
- **Cold-water fish:** Mackerel, salmon and sardines are all great sources of omega-3 fatty acids. Salmon also contains astaxanthin, a carotenoid with anti-inflammatory properties that can also improve skin elasticity.
- **Free-range eggs:** The most complete food! Eggs are an awesome source of protein as well, and they help to repair cells that have suffered free-radical damage from pollution and poor diet. Eat them poached, scrambled, folded or in an omelette. Always serve with some veggies, too.
- **Natural organic dairy:** Rich in vitamin B2 (riboflavin), vitamin B12 and vitamin B5. Riboflavin is necessary for cell growth and regeneration,

and protects skin cells from oxidative damage. Add fresh goat's cheese to salads, mix Greek yoghurt and honey as a dessert, or mix in with fresh mint and olive oil as a yoghurt dip.

dairy: dos and don'ts

Dairy can be good for some people. It contains B vitamins, which aid cell metabolism and growth, giving you glowing skin and reduced blemishes.

There is good cheese and bad cheese; stick to fresh cheeses like goat's cheese, feta and mozzarella. Avoid processed cheese, and anything that looks too dyed and contains preservatives and flavourings. And if it's peelable . . . bin it.

Even with fresh cheese, though, don't go too mad – but a little sprinkle of goat's cheese in your salad is a lovely addition.

TOP TIP: Order a cheese platter over a sugary dessert when out for dinner.

When it comes to milk, opt for organic full-fat (from cows, goats or sheep). Buying organic is important! It is loaded with more omega-3 fatty acids and vitamins than other milk.

If you find dairy doesn't work for you, swap it for some almond milk, rice milk, oat milk, coconut milk or coconut yoghurt instead.

why did fat get such a bad rep?

Well the problem with fat is that people label it all the same. But, as you now know, not all fats are bad!

The ones to watch out for are trans fats. These can clog the arteries, release free radicals into the body and cause inflammation, making you both fat and toxic. They occur in many processed and ready-to-eat foods, diet foods, margarine, processed meats and hydrogenated oils. Trans fats increase the shelf life of foods, but can contribute to obesity, cancer, heart disease and infertility.

switch your mindset

This new way of eating is all about crowding in, rather than cutting out.

Your skin is a reflection of your internals; it always reveals when you are eating well. You can absolutely eat your way to glowing skin; all you need to do is pack in the good stuff.

Here is a list of my top skin-glowing foods:

- **Red peppers:** These are amazing sources of vitamin C, which helps regulate the structural protein collagen, keeping your skin taut and toned. Cut them up for a snack, or throw them in stir-fries or salads.

- **Chia seeds**: Super-rich in omega-3s and calcium. If you're a veggie, make sure you get some of these into you! They soak up ten times their weight in water, and hydrate your body to give you glowing, dewy skin. Sprinkle them over your salads or yoghurt for a bit of crunch and texture, or make my Three-Ingredient Banana Chia Pudding (see page 93).
- **Brazil nuts**: These contain the amazing trace mineral selenium, which helps to protect the skin from cell damage. Sadly, due to our overworked soils, we don't have much selenium in our diet, but just two of these nuts will load your body up with your daily dose. You can also pop them into your morning smoothie or brekkie bowl.
- **Liver**: Yes, liver. It's an amazing source of vitamin A (and other fat-soluble vitamins). Vitamin A promotes cell turnover and gives you healthy skin. Liver isn't something you can find easily, but ask your butcher. You can sauté it in some spices and coconut oil and then pop it into salads. It tastes delicious, I promise.
- **Kale**: Head cheerleader for a reason, this veggie is an excellent source of iron, vitamin C and sulphur. Sulphur is necessary for collagen synthesis (which falls short as we age). Sauté some kale with a side of eggs in the morning, or steam it with some fish for a sumptuous supper.
- **Oysters**: A little bit fancy, these delicacies provide a super source of zinc – an essential mineral that plays a role in your immune function, protein synthesis and cell division. It protects the skin from UV radiation and acts as an anti-inflammatory agent. A more budget-friendly option for zinc is a handful of pumpkin seeds.

Look at it as an exciting adventure as you introduce all these new foods into your diet. You will be so spoilt for choice that you won't have time for junk food. This positive mindset will help you every step of the way.

eating out

This six-week plan isn't really a diet – it's a lifestyle. I want you to take it seriously, but it also has to fit in around you. So of course you can eat out – don't be a hermit, enjoy yourself! Just choose the cleanest meal possible:

- **Avoid added sugar and hidden sugars**: Steer clear of dishes that include the words caramelised, glazed, BBQ sauce, or sweet and sour.

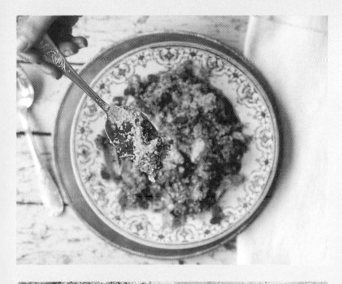

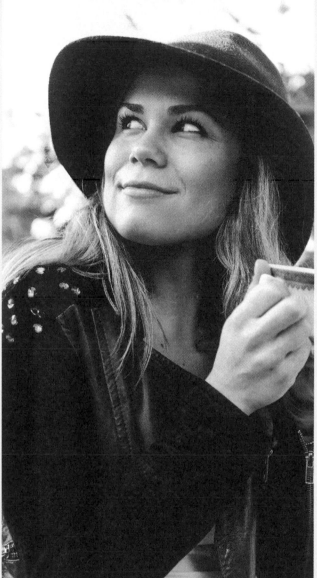

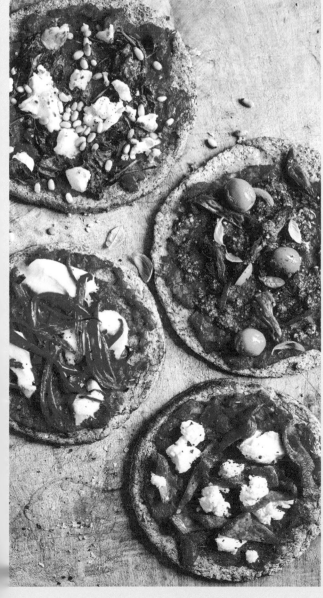

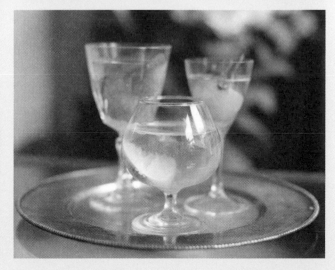

- **Pass on the bread basket**: If it sits there in front of you, you will be sure to grab a bite.
- **Substitute when you order**: Swap chips for steamed vegetables, or have a side salad instead of bread.
- **Dress your own salad**: Most salad dressings contain added sugar, so opt for no dressing but ask for some olive oil so you can dress your own.
- **Think simple**: The best choices include fish of the day, a good roast, veggies or a fresh salad.

Restaurants tend to be very accommodating these days, so don't be afraid to ask for alternatives. Aim to get your plate mainly consisting of a nice bit of delicious protein, healthy fats and some fresh veg.

Q&A

Q: Is soy milk OK?

A: No. Whatever you do, please ditch the soy milk. Often my clients smile with pride when they tell me they've switched to soy milk lattes, as we are constantly told that soy is good for us. The problem is that soy milk doesn't resemble traditional soy found in Asian cultures in the slightest. There it is consumed in the form of miso, tempeh, natto and soy sauce, which have been fermented. This fermentation process breaks down the phytic acid – but soy milk contains copious amount of this acid. Phytic acid is present in the outer portion of all seeds, and blocks the absorption of essential minerals such as calcium, magnesium, iron and zinc in particular – meaning all your good work in getting these minerals into your system is being undone! So switch to organic milk, rice milk, oat milk, nut milk or make my Almond Milk (see page 261) or Coconut Milk (see page 258) instead.

Q: I have the biggest energy slump at 4pm – how can I combat this?
A: Quitting sugar and introducing fat is going to help to stabilise your blood sugar levels. So it should help you to get off that rollercoaster of highs and lows during the day. However, that 4pm slump can still kick in, so the trick is to have healthy snacks on hand – like an apple with nut butter, half an avocado, a handful of nuts or a green juice. It's good to change your space when your energy is low: go for a walk, do a lap of the office, make yourself a herbal tea or grab a coconut water.

Q: I feel like I need something sweet after a meal, just to satisfy my taste buds. What do I do?
A: I know this feeling! I suggest you opt for something wholesome, like toasted coconut flakes, a handful of cinnamon-toasted nuts or some berries with coconut yoghurt. My lifesaver is peppermint and liquorice tea. Liquorice root not only tastes super-sweet – combating your cravings – it also feeds the adrenal glands, reducing stress.

Q: Am I intolerant to dairy?
A: The best way to know whether you are allergic or intolerant to something is to remove it from your diet for two weeks. See how you feel, then reintroduce it after two weeks. Your body will react if it's intolerant, and if you feel OK then you are probably fine with it. Quite a lot of this is about using your intuition; you can best tell what your body likes and doesn't. Week 4 of this programme is about healing the digestive system to help cure intolerances and beat that bloated feeling.

Q: I never have enough time to be healthy. How do you do it?
A: I've had clients who are the CEO of multinationals, and busy working mums without a moment to spare. I've seen it all. It's all about preparation – use Sunday to plan ahead. Make my Smoky Roast Chicken with Sweet Potato Wedges (see page 188), Green Queen Quinoa Dish (see page 179) and Raw Chocolate Balls (see page 102) for the coming week ahead. Also, take a look at my Speedy Suppers section – this chapter was made for you.

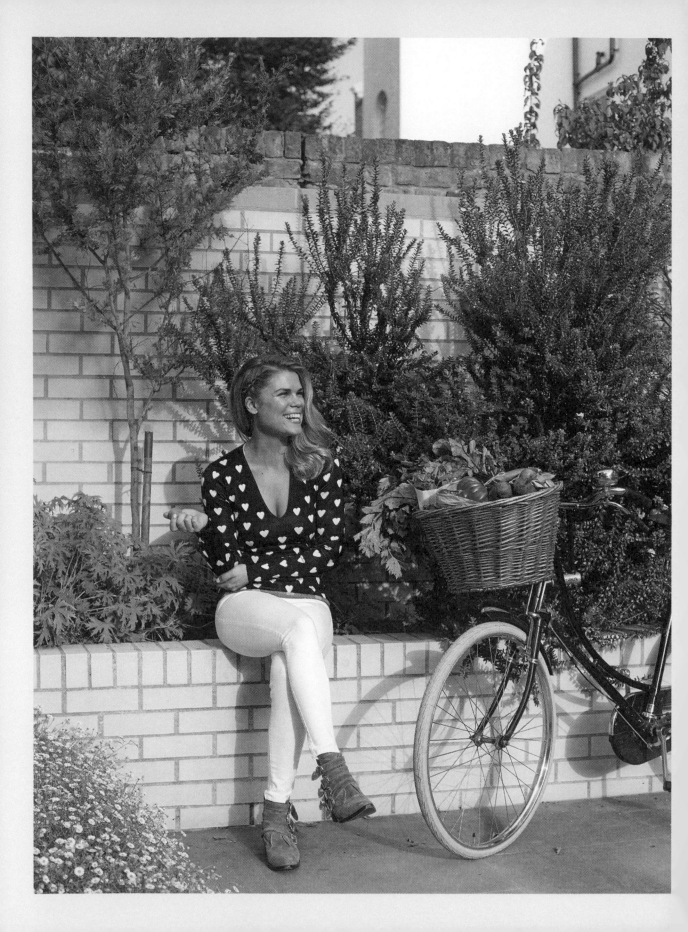

EAT

clean,

THINK

clean

week three

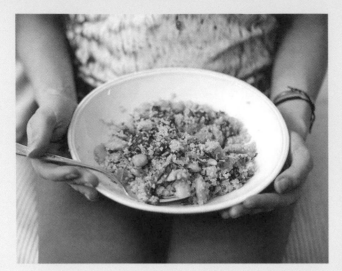

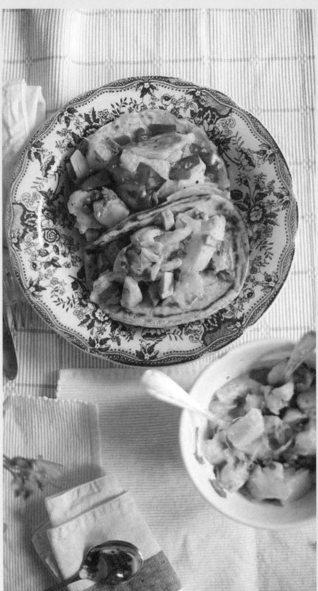

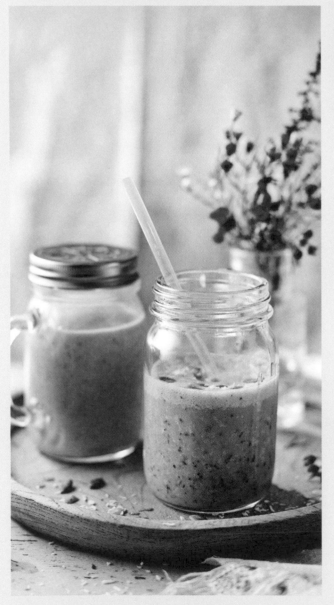

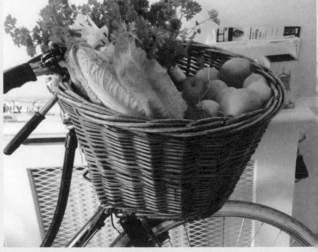

Eating clean goes hand in hand with thinking clean. *Get the Glow* isn't just for six weeks – it's about the amazing person you will be for life.

self-love

We have talked a lot about food so far, but this week is all about how you think. I want you to fall back in love with yourself! To truly love every inch of you.

This may sound silly and a little esoteric, but hear me out . . . Every muscle in the body needs to be used daily to grow and function properly. This is the same with self-love. To really fall back in love with yourself you need to commit to being kind to yourself everyday. First I want you to write down all the negative things you say to yourself on a daily basis. We all do it . . . be honest.

I will help you out. I'm talking about thoughts like:

I am too fat. I look dreadful today. I hate my body. My skin is terrible.

Imagine if your best friend or loved one said this to you. Well, frankly, you wouldn't want them to be part of your life. So why do you tell yourself these things? And of course, negative thoughts impact on other areas of life too.

I never have enough money. I am so unlucky in love. I hate my job.

The problem is, we focus our energy on negativity and pain, which isn't good for us. The relationship you have with yourself is precious, so it is essential to start flexing your self-love muscle.

So let's begin!

positive affirmations

Your first step is to use positive affirmations. Don't roll your eyes – these do work!

A belief is something you say to yourself over and over; we can change the way we think by mastering our thoughts. So every morning, I want you to tell yourself three positive things that you like about yourself. These can be related to your body, or your life circumstances.

If you don't know where to start, how about reversing the negative thoughts you may have about yourself? Or try this affirmation:

I live, love and learn every day.

I like to say my positive affirmations in the shower before I start the day . . . along with a good sing-song.

Continue this exercise everyday, and just like brushing your teeth it will become an ingrained habit. Then sit back and watch your confidence sparkle. And remember that positive vibes create positive lives!

don't compare . . . congratulate!

We are a nation obsessed with celebrities; we love to watch their highs, and especially their lows. It makes us feel less alone in our own flaws. But other people's shortcomings don't really make our lives any better.

Neither is lusting after what others have a good use of our time. Comparing yourself to friends – whether it's their clothes, body shape, wealth or beauty – can make you feel inadequate, different and isolated.

Instead, stop comparing yourself, and start loving your amazing body.

Try congratulating, rather than comparing. Give that person a compliment on their outfit, hair, skin or circumstances, even if it's just in your head. This change will make you feel connected and happy, and will attract more praise your way.

In truth, the other person is looking right back at you comparing themselves to you, so why not break down those boundaries?

you are not alone

No one is perfect. I don't always look at my body and think 'yes!' However, what has really changed for me is that I don't dwell on it; I don't pity myself or bathe in negativity.

So when you're feeling negative and down, don't reach for the ice cream or starve yourself. Promise me that you'll do something positive instead – like go for a walk, have a delicious nutritious snack, call a friend or buy a new lipstick – spoil yourself with love, and focus on all that is good and positive in your life.

We are all on a journey, and writing this book is part of my journey; it's part of my healing. Don't wait to figure life out, just get on with living it.

be authentic

Unhappiness often comes from not feeling understood. If we are true to ourselves and behave and act as we really are, then we feel connected to our sense of self.

The problem is we often lie to ourselves, creating a false image to make others like us. Being authentic is the key to happiness.

be happy in the moment

We all put off happiness. You know the thoughts: *Once I lose weight, meet the guy, get the perfect job . . . I'll be happy.*

But if we can't be happy in this moment, with what we have right now, how on earth are we going to happy in the future?

I used to be a runner (sadly not the marathon kind); I used to run away from situations. Whenever something got tough, I would leave – I'd change job, change friends, even change country. I thought that I would find happiness somewhere else; that someone else would fix me, change me and make my life better. I soon realised that a state of peace and completeness could only come from within. It isn't something we learn overnight, but practising clean thoughts will help you fall back in love with yourself.

I know I am getting a little hippy on you, but I'm just trying to teach you that your attitude is so important.

The following simple steps will help you create more happiness in your life.

- **Affirm:** Repeat your positive affirmations every day.
- **Help others:** Start spreading the love and feel it bounce back.
- **Treat yourself:** Give yourself gifts; they can be tiny like a bubble bath, magazine or pedicure, or curl up with a book.
- **Get social:** Surround yourself with people you love and who light you up.
- **Talk it out:** Whatever you're going through, don't face it alone; talk to your friends or family.
- **Nourish:** Feed your body with healthy food that you love.
- **Get active:** Move your body every day to help produce serotonin, the happy hormone.
- **Give gratitude:** Write down everything that is going well in your life, and reflect on all the wonders you have.
- **Smile big:** It actually makes you feel happier.
- **Think positive:** You can do it!

Q&A

Q: But I hate my body – how can I love it?
A: Like you learned to ride a bike, you will learn to love yourself. You will get up and fall off, but eventually you will get on and stay on. You may even become brave enough to take your hands off the handlebars! Just practise the steps above and trust that it will come.

Q: I feel like my healthy lifestyle is making me antisocial. My friends keep saying I'm boring; what do I do?
A: Living healthily doesn't mean you can't go out or spend time with your friends. It just means you may socialise in a few different ways – why not go to a yoga class, or go out for brunch instead of a boozy night out? If your friends aren't being supportive of your life change, then perhaps it's time to branch out and widen your circle of pals. I've made a lot of new, like-minded friends at fitness classes and wellness events.

Q: I'm an emotional eater. Please help!
A: Don't walk through the door and reach for the cupboards – food is not a distraction. Instead, stay away from the kitchen – hop in the shower, read a book, close your eyes and take a breath. Combat stress with love, not food.

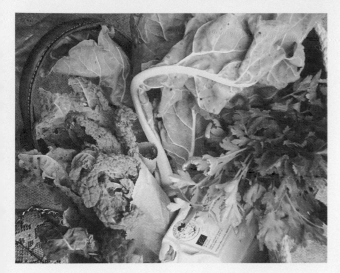

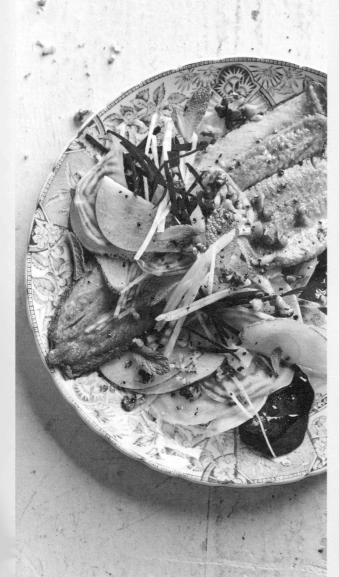

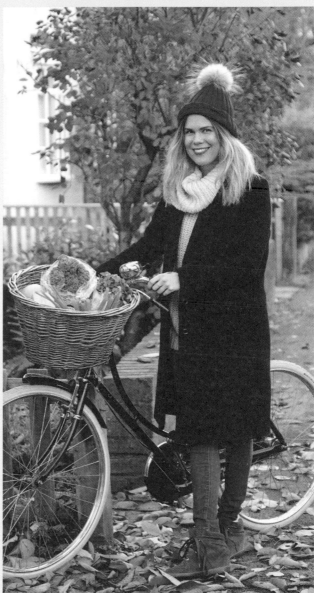

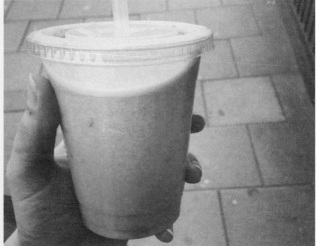

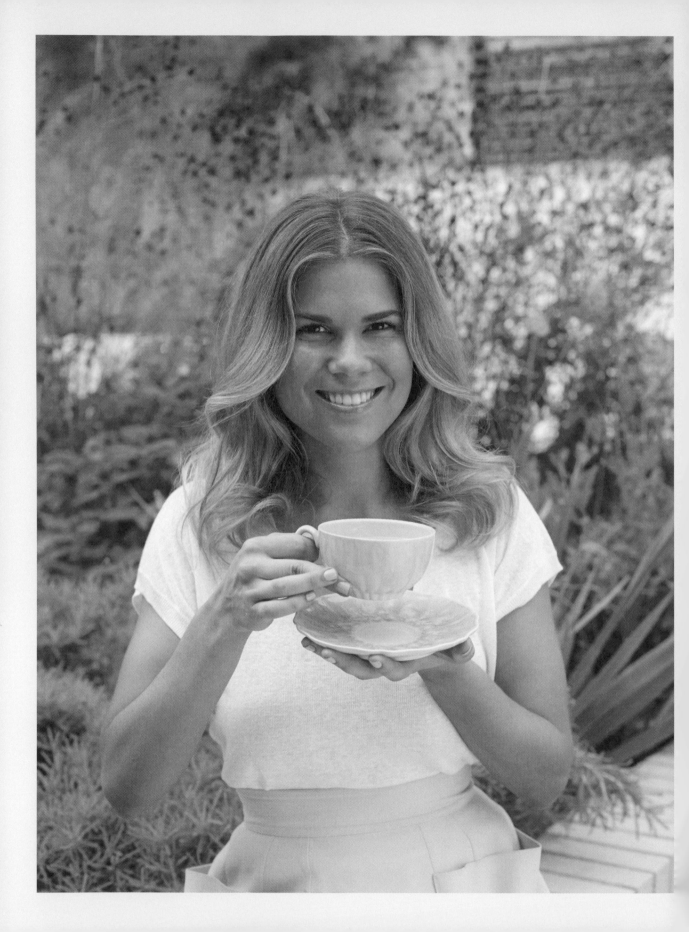

BEAT
the
BLOAT

week four

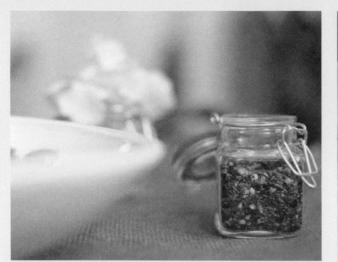
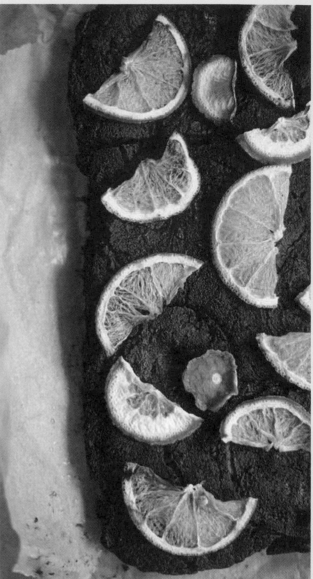
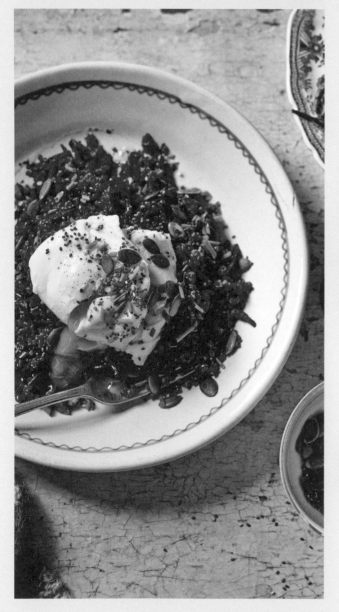
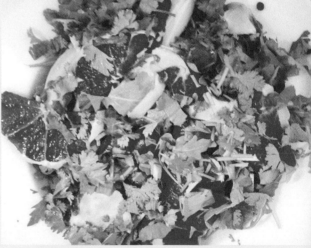

So you're eating and thinking clean, you're sugar free and nourishing your body with good food. Give yourself a pat on the back! Now we're going to create healthy internals to beat that bloated feeling.

get acquainted with your gut

Gut health isn't a sexy subject, but your digestive system is so important. After all, it's where you absorb your food – and your gut contains about 70 per cent of your immune system, which is a lot! When your gut lining is damaged it allows partially digested foods to slip through and escape into your bloodstream. This puts great strain on your liver (which detoxifies the blood) and this in turn stresses the body every time you eat. So even if you eat all the kale and coconuts in the world, you'll never reach optimum health with an unhealthy gut.

Many things can damage the state of your gut, with oral contraceptives, alcohol, sugar and stress being just a handful of harmful factors. But I know you can't necessarily wave a magic wand and banish these from your life, so in five easy steps I'll show you how to keep bad digestion at bay.

1. goodbye gluten!

The first step is to say good riddance to gluten. You may have noticed that my recipes are very low in carbohydrates, with no bread in sight, and they're also always gluten free.

This is because gluten can cause a huge amount of inflammation in the gut, which leads to bloating, poor digestion and even inflammatory disease if consumed on a regular basis.

what is gluten?

Gluten is a protein found in wheat, rye

and barley. The most important glutinous grain to ditch is wheat, which is like sandpaper for the gut.

When there is an excess of gluten, gluten phytates bind with calcium, iron, magnesium and phosphorus – making these minerals harder for your body to absorb effectively, leaving you deprived. When these minerals are lacking you can feeling sluggish and low in energy.

Not everyone is gluten intolerant, and I don't think you have to give it up forever, but most people see an improvement when they reduce it in their diet.

After just a few weeks, you'll enjoy:
- More energy
- Less bloating
- Better digestion

Sounds pretty wonderful, right? Try going gluten free for the next two weeks, and see what a difference it can make.

life without gluten

On a very basic level, a gluten-free life means no bread, takeaway pizza, pasta and no to most cookies and cakes. I know this sounds a little bleak, but there are lots of great alternatives as you'll see from the recipes in the next section of the book.

gluten-free goodness

With these simple swaps, you'll soon find that going gluten free is as easy as 1, 2, 3!

swap this:	for this:
pizza	cauliflower pizza (see page 204)
white bread	my quinoa bread (see page 96)
couscous	millet
white flour	buckwheat flour or ground almonds in baking
pasta	courgette ribbons

I know it's hard to part ways with these carbs. They're comforting, but soon you'll feel so amazing without them that you will forget toast ever existed!

watch out, gluten's about

Gluten can be hiding sneakily in many foods that you might not expect:
- Soups
- Condiments
- Alcohol
- Breadcrumbs

- Hot dogs
- Salad dressings
- Stock cubes
- Processed foods
- Gravy
- Barley, bulghur, spelt

2. beneficial bacteria

The second step to help you beat the bloat is to restore the balance between the good and bad bacteria in your gut.

Although it sounds unpleasant, bacteria are the foundation of your life and health. Imbalanced bacteria in the gut causes digestive issues, low immunity, weight gain and skin problems. Good bacteria are essential for your health, as they:

- extract energy from food
- modulate the immune system
- help regulate hormones.

fab fermented foods

The best way to restore this imbalance is to get probiotic-rich food into your diet. Foods that have been fermented are rich in enzymes that help you digest and absorb food.

- **Sauerkraut**: Fermented cabbage
- **Kefir**: Fermented yoghurt
- **Kombucha**: Fermented tea
- **Miso**: Fermented soy beans

action plan

You should aim to eat some form of fermented food every day for the next two weeks. It is best to get good bacteria into the gut through a food source (rather than tons of yoghurt drinks) as your body will absorb it better.

So, try to eat 2 tablespoons of kefir or sauerkraut per day, with meals. Ideally choose unpasteurised sauerkraut or kefir, as these contain the highest amounts of good bacteria (the pasteurisation kills a lot of it).

Doubling up with probiotic tablets – which are a concentrated form of good bacteria – will also help restore the gut to its natural healthy state. They particularly help with IBS, constipation and diarrhoea. Every morning, take the recommended daily allowance of probiotics, making sure you choose a probiotic that contains at least 4 billion viable organisms with as many different types of probiotic species as possible, from both the lactobacillus and bifidobacterium families.

3. pro protein

Protein is the third step to beat the bloat. It is key to living a hot and healthy life, and it helps heal your gut too. Protein contains anti-inflammatory omega-3 fats that soothe the gut lining. It helps to build strong hair, promote glowing skin and maintain steady blood-sugar levels, as it is metabolised over a long period of time. So make sure you include it in every meal.

It is best to get protein from animal sources, as they contain all eight essential amino acids; however, there are lots of awesome veggie and vegan options too. Variety is key, so take a look at this list of the best sources of protein:

- Grass-fed/pasture-raised meat
- Wild game
- Free-range chicken and turkey
- Cold-water fish
- Seafood
- Free-range eggs
- Hemp seeds
- Chia seeds
- Quinoa
- Superfoods – spirulina and wild blue-green algae
- Pumpkin seeds
- Pulses and beans – make sure these are soaked overnight before being eaten to promote proper digestion

grass-fed meat

Many people think meat is unhealthy and that you should limit your meat intake. I totally respect that people don't eat meat for ethical reasons, and others don't like the taste. But if you aren't vegetarian, meat is a good protein source and therefore an extremely important part of your diet. Of course, I'm not saying you should eat frankfurters all day long, but good-quality grass-fed meat is very beneficial to your beautiful body.

'Grass-fed meat' simply means that the animal has eaten grass its entire life. You are probably thinking that cows always eat grass . . . well, not all of them. In fact, some of the beef on supermarket shelves comes from cows placed in massive pens and stuffed full of grain, as it's a lot cheaper than rotating them around grass fields.

It's common sense that what goes into the cow will go into you once you've devoured your delicious beef stew. Omega-3 fatty acids originate from the green leaves of plants and algae, so grass-fed animals have more of these essential nutrients due to their diet. In the same way, fish contain copious amounts of omega-3 fatty acids due to their algae and phytoplankton-rich diets. Omega-3 fatty acids reduce inflammation in the body, improve brain function – and enhance your glow.

grass-fed goodness

- Grass-fed meat contains 20 times more vitamin E than corn- or soy-fed meat.

- It doesn't contain any nasty trans fatty acids.
- It is the richest known natural source of CLA (conjugated linoleic acid), which makes you slimmer.
- It contains extra amounts of beta-carotene, a powerful antioxidant.

Switching to grass-fed isn't a fad or a new diet, it's just eating proper food. So cut out processed ham, sausages and fast-food meat and hunt down a good butcher or order your meat online from a farm. It really isn't more expensive, and you don't have to eat it every day. It tastes so much better, and you will seriously feel the benefits.

4. beat the bloat with bone broth

Going gluten free, and introducing good bacteria and quality protein into your diet will have done wonders for your gut health. My last tip is to drink bone broth.

This may sound a little odd and out-dated, but hear me out. Drinking bone broth is an amazing ancient technique for restoring your gut to good health. Bone broth is similar to stock, and we all know that chicken stock can cure a cold.

- The gelatin found in bone broth is a hydrophilic colloid, helping to support proper digestion.
- It contains easily absorbable calcium, magnesium, phosphorus, silicon, sulphur and trace minerals.
- It reduces inflammation in the body.
- The gelatin also promotes healthy hair and nail growth.

For those who suffer with terrible digestion, I recommend drinking one to two cups of bone broth a day.

how to make bone broth

- 500g grass-fed beef bones (or other animal bones)
- 1 white onion, roughly chopped
- 2 bay leaves
- 2 tsp sea salt
- 4 tbsp cider vinegar

Wash your bones in warm water. Place them in a large stock pot, or your biggest pot. Cover the tops of the bones with water. Put the onion in the water, along with the rest of the ingredients. Bring to the boil, then reduce to a very low heat and simmer for 4–6 hours. Strain the broth through a sieve and put it in containers. The broth is freezable, so divide it up and keep some for a later date.

Use in soups, to sauté veggies or to drink before meals.

5. more ways to beat the bloat

You now have all the foundations to aid your digestion and heal your gut. Here are some more quick tips, if you need a little extra boost:

- Take amino acid L-glutamine, aloe vera, slippery elm and magnesium citrate.
- Drink a cup of camomile, liquorice root or peppermint tea; these soothe and relax the belly.
- Give your tummy a massage in a clockwise circular motion to start moving everything around.
- Take belly breaths – breathe deeply into your belly; inhale for three counts and exhale for four counts. This calms the nervous system and gets blood pumping around the digestive system.
- Add a teaspoon of apple cider vinegar to your water before you eat; this will get your digestion going.
- Get some sunshine: vitamin D helps regulate your immune system, crowds out pathogens and regulates the microbiomes.

Q&A

Q: How much protein should I eat?
A: Aim for a fist-size of protein in all of your meals. Mix up the sources to keep it interesting, and always eat foods you love – for example, don't force-feed yourself fish if you don't like it. This is all about enjoyment, not punishment.

Q: Can you have too many eggs?
A: Yes, you can overdo any food. Our bodies love variety, so just stick to two eggs three times a week.

Q: Where can I find probiotics and fermented foods?
A: Your local health food store, a chemist, or online.

Q: If something is labelled as 'gluten free', does this mean it's OK?
A: Not always. Many gluten-free products are pumped full of chemicals trying to replicate the gluten. Stick to breads made from rice, buckwheat, quinoa or millet flour. If you're not gluten intolerant, rye or spelt are also great options. As a rule of thumb, look for bread with the fewest ingredients or make your own.

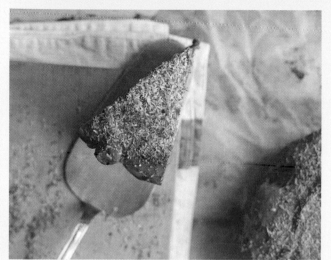

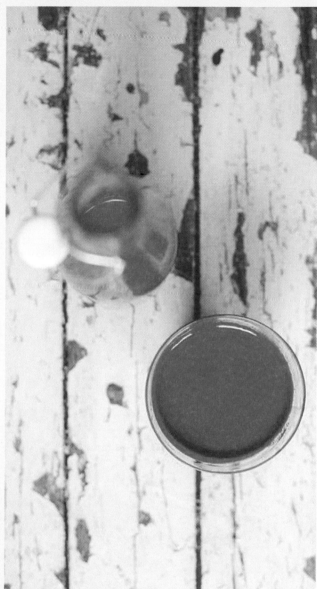

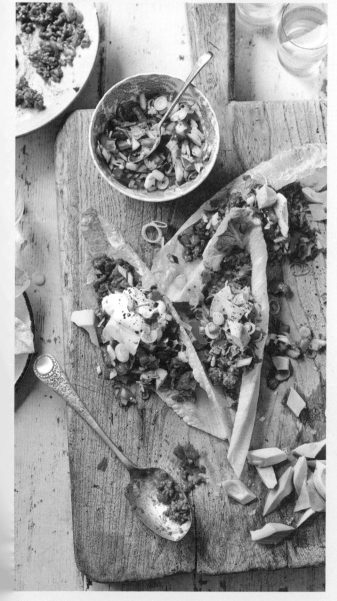

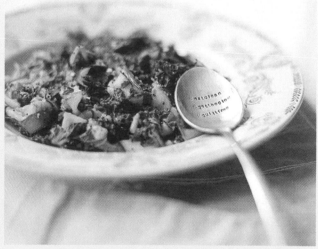

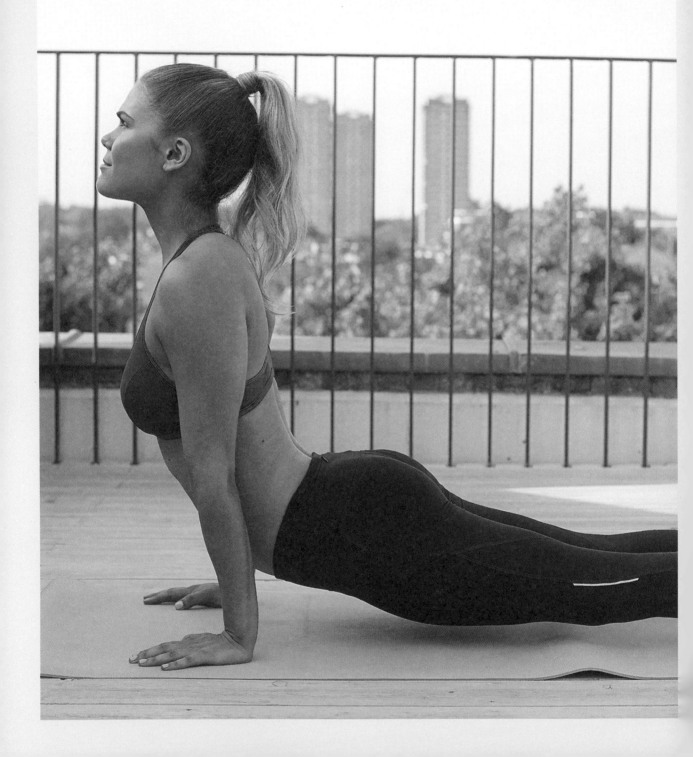

REST

and

DIGEST

week five

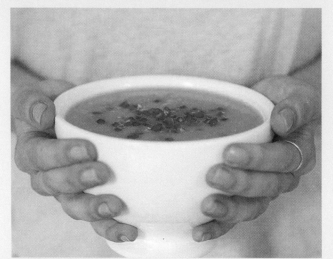

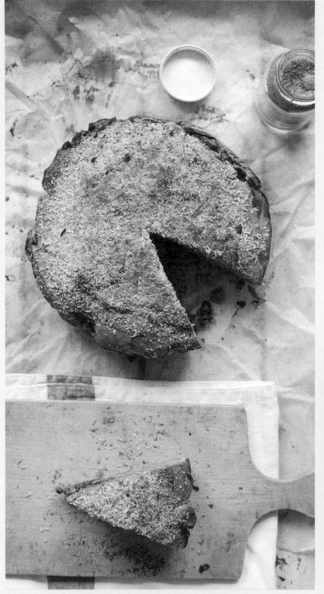

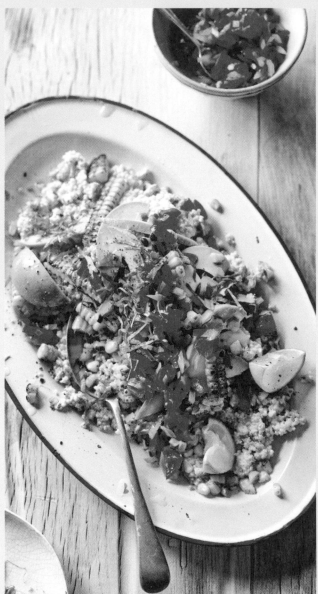

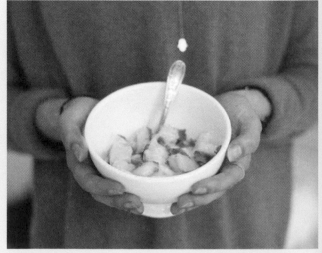

Stress not only affects your mind, but also your waistline, digestion and overall well-being. This week I will show you how to say goodbye to stress to enable the hottest, healthiest and happiest you.

mindful eating

It not just about what you eat but how you eat. Eating mindfully is a very important part of getting the glow. It allows you to savour every morsel of your food, meaning you will eat less, feel fuller, reduce bloating and digest food more quickly.

We live life fast: we eat on the go, standing up, in front of the computer, and hardly ever at the table. Most of us are overstressed, overtired and over-worked, which often leads us to mind-lessly shove bad food into our mouths and make poor lifestyle choices.

When we eat on the go we are in a state of 'fight or flight', meaning our blood is directed to our muscles instead of going to the digestive system where it is needed. We should sit down mindfully with our meals and switch to a state of rest and digest. This is the sweet spot.

Mindfulness isn't just about how you eat, but is about being conscious in everything we do. It helps us to get out of our heads and into our hearts. Reduced mind chatter certainly makes for happier and healthier living.

how to eat mindfully

- **Eat at a table**: Not standing up.
- **Turn off any distractions**: No TV, computer, phone or work. This helps you feel fuller and more connected to your food as you concentrate on what is on your plate, not on the screen.
- **Chew your food**: Your body works hard to draw all the nutrients out of your food, so help yourself by chewing 10 times before you swallow. This will make you eat less,

feel full quicker, and vanquish that post-dinner bulge.

· **Wait 20 minutes to get seconds**: It takes a while to feel full, so you might not actually need that extra portion.

· **Take breaths between mouthfuls**: Don't wolf it down, enjoy it! Taking your time allows you to appreciate your food and enjoy its taste and texture.

meditation

If you are like me and seem to be always in your head, thinking, worrying and daydreaming, meditation may be the key to your happiness. There has been lots of exciting research into the notion that the gut is our second brain. With 100,000 neurotransmitters lining the length of the gut, it really is quite sensitive. The brain and gut are connected by the vagus nerve, which travels from the base of the brain to the gut. If your digestive system is out of whack, pain signals are sent up to the brain. When you put life's stresses on top of this . . . all hell breaks loose. Therefore calming the mind helps calm the gut.

For me mediation was the final factor that helped heal my digestive problems and stop stress taking over my life.

Meditation is about training the mind to be conscious. It is a great tool to help you become present. Most of the time we live worrying about the future or reliving the past. Meditation allows you to be present and enjoy the moment, as well as these other benefits:

· It helps reduce stress
· It relaxes the body and mind
· It makes you feel calmer and happier.

how does meditation work?

There are numerous ways to meditate. Some people do yoga, t'ai chi, dancing or painting to get out of their heads and into their bodies. The most well-known form, though, is seated meditation.

To do this, find a quiet place where you feel comfortable, and turn off all distractions. Sit on a chair, or on the floor with your legs crossed, and close your eyes.

Inhale for three counts, then slowly exhale for four counts. Breathe into your belly not into your chest – this helps calm your nervous system. Feel your belly rise and fall. Repeat this ten times, keeping your eyes closed and your mind focused on your breathing. Try not to let your mind wander. If it does, just come back to counting your breaths. When you're finished, slowly bring yourself back into the present and see how much better you feel.

Try meditating every day for a week, and at the end of the seven days look back to see how much calmer you feel. Start by mediating for a minute, then slowly add on another until you are able to sit calmly for around 20 minutes. Make this part of your routine, and don't let things get in the way. You can always make time to meditate: do it between meetings, on the train or before bed. There is always space in the day to be still.

work it out

When I lived in Sydney I was so inspired by the attitude people had to exercise. It was a way of life, a social engagement. There was no laziness about it; people would get up at 5am to catch the first wave.

I wasn't into exercise growing up, and I've never liked the gym, but daily movement has not only built up my booty but has given me boundless energy and helped me to manage stress.

I find it's best to exercise in the morning – that way it's done, and no last-minute work crisis or social engagement will get in the way. Pop your gym bag by the door and commit to a class with a friend – buddying up will help you turn up! Put it in your diary just as you would an appointment you can't miss;

treating it with importance will make sure it gets done.

If you can't afford a gym subscription, commit to a walk, go for a quick jog or even do a free aerobics class on YouTube! Don't make excuses . . . you can do it.

replenish your reserves

Quite a lot of us push ourselves in the gym. It is therefore super-important that we replenish our reserves afterwards, so we can get up and do it again tomorrow. What you should eat post-workout depends on what exercise you did.

- **High-intensity cardio workouts:** Stick to healthy fats and proteins. Make my Strong and Lean Smoothie (see page 255), Scrambled Eggs with Pesto and Avocado (see page 72) or Smoked Salmon and Fattoush Salad with Avocado Mash (see page 149).
- **Lifting weights:** It's better to have more carbs post-workout, but stick to things like my Sweet Potato Dip (see page 110), Green Queen Quinoa Dish (see page 179) or one of my Post-Workout Balls (see page 103).

Try not to exercise on a full stomach, as it takes your body a few hours to digest food. I like to have a smoothie or juice before a session, as smoothies and juices can be absorbed quickly by the body. Coffee is also a great pre-workout drink as it is packed with antioxidants. Don't abuse it, though, and only use it if you're training in the morning.

soak, stroke and sleep away the stress

A great way to reduce stress is to have a soak in a delicious warm Epsom salt bath. Epsom salts help relax the muscles and ease you into a good night's sleep. Just pour 1 cup of Epsom salts into a bath and soak in the tub for 15 minutes. This is great for recovering post-workout, too, as it eases tired muscles.

I also love dry brushing before getting into a bath or shower; it's the best way to get rid of stubborn areas of cellulite and to eliminate toxic build-up from the body. So since we've ditched the junk from our diet, it's time to brush it out of the system too.

how to dry brush

Grab a natural bristle brush. Before you hop in the shower brush it over your bare skin, starting from your toes and moving towards your head. Brush in an upward sweeping motion (be careful around sensitive areas), and give that butt a good go too.

benefits of dry body brushing

- Improves muscle tone
- Evens out fat deposits
- Regulates body temperature
- Stimulates hormones and oil-producing glands, making your skin glow
- Blasts cellulite

sleep sweetly

Sleep is key to a healthy body. It helps banish sugar cravings, reduces hunger and banishes stress. Aim to sleep from 10pm to 6am – this is the best time to be in bed to allow your body to restore itself. Here are some tips on how to have a good night's sleep:

- Don't eat after 8.30pm and get in bed for 10pm.
- Have a small chamomile tea before bed.
- Limit alcohol.
- Wind down and de-stress before bed.
- Avoid any screen time before bed; try reading instead.
- Make your room dark and cold with cosy bedding.

Q&A

Q: I struggle with portion control – how can I combat overeating?

A: Mindfulness is the key to overcoming this. Slow down, chew your food and you'll soon find you won't be reaching for more. As a general rule, per meal I would aim for a fist-size of protein, the same for grains or starchy veg, and then an unlimited amount of non-starchy veg. Try and eat one big plateful and then not have any more.

When you serve yourself, try not to have lots of extras lying around on the table. Imagine you're eating in a restaurant – you'd never ask for a second helping when eating out!

Q: What time should I eat in the evening?

A: The timing of food does matter; it's best to eat your biggest meal for lunch and a lighter one for dinner, as your digestive fire burns much lower in the evening. Aim to eat before 8pm so your food is properly digested before you hit the hay.

Q: I'm feeling run-down – what should I take?

A: Boost your immune system with this little concoction. Boil the kettle and pour the water into a mug. Crush in 1 garlic clove, add 1 tablespoon honey, 1 tablespoon freshly grated ginger and ½ teaspoon whole cloves, then let it sit for 5 minutes and drink. Repeat three times a day.

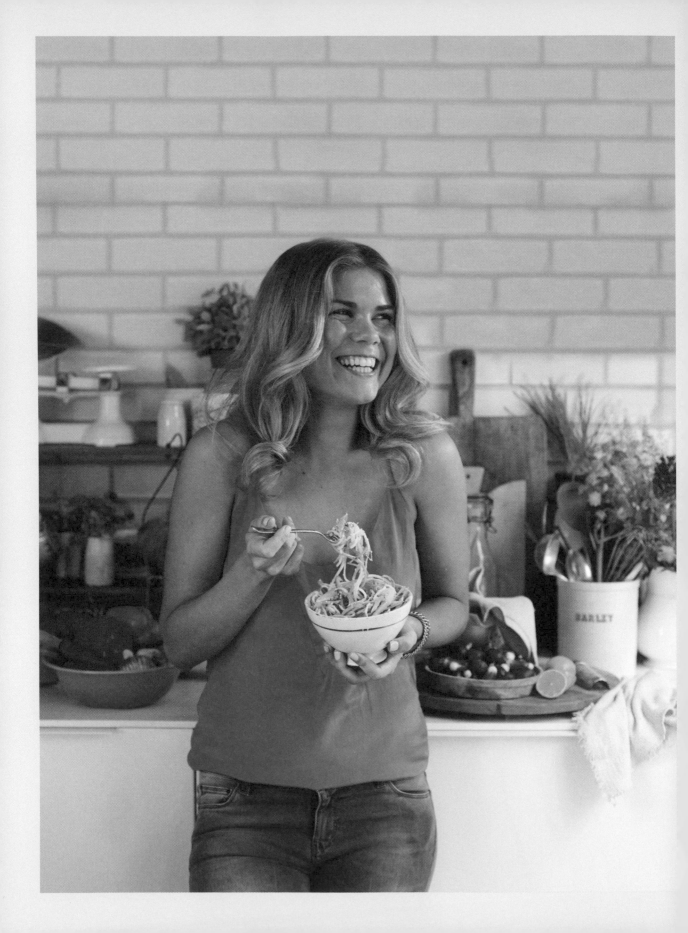

LIVE

your

GLOW

week six

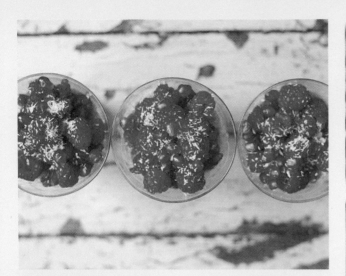

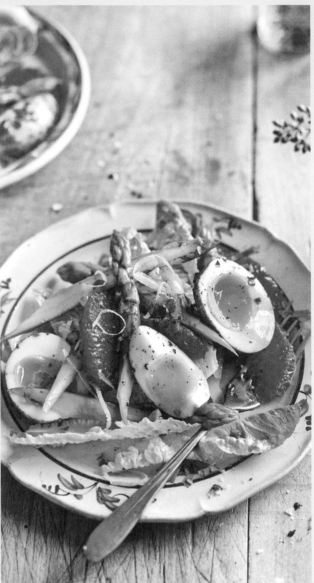

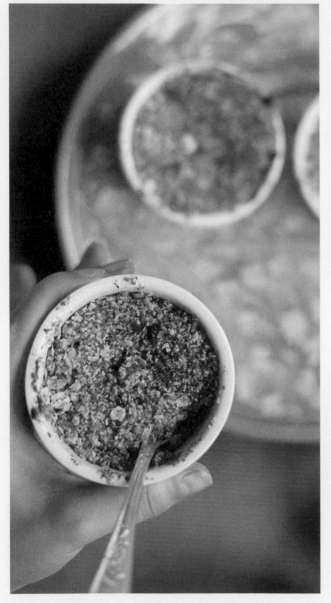

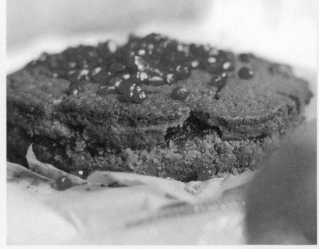

Congratulations – you are in your final week!
Now it's time to set you up with healthy habits to
ensure you live your glow . . . for life.

post-programme binge

Now you are nearing the end, it doesn't mean you can swerve back to your old ways and overindulge on sugar and bad carbs. I'm not saying you can't ever have these naughty treats, but you should eat consciously and because you love it, not as an act of anger, sadness or boredom.

I think the best time to eat something naughty is when you're out to dinner.

Why?

Well, unless you are at a buffet there is only one piece of pie: when it's gone, it's gone. The restaurant setting makes you savour the taste and enjoy the experience so much more than you would a giant tub of vanilla ice cream while sitting on your sofa.

a word about sabotage . . .

You may have noticed a few pesky friends or colleagues trying to lead you astray over the past 6 weeks, tempting you with cake or big nights out.

This is totally normal and to be expected. Sometimes people see others changing around them and they feel threatened, so they try to sabotage your decisions.

Be aware of this, and use the tools you've learned over the past 6 weeks – being mindful of what you're eating, and your reasons for embarking on this programme in the first place.

avoid the snack-trap

And of course, we're often our own saboteur. We've all been there – we've eaten healthily all day but have blown it by snacking on treats the moment we're home. Stop this by:

- having a big cup of herbal tea as soon as you're through the door
- spending the evening with friends
- staying out of the kitchen and not opening the fridge door
- having a green juice – it's packed full of nutrients to satisfy your cravings
- eating a proper lunch – so many people don't eat enough for this crucial meal
- drinking a glass of water – that rumble in your stomach might be because you're thirsty.

Snacking constantly is very taxing for your digestive system; leave gaps between your meals so your body can rest and digest.

running low on the glow?

It could be that you're falling into the snack trap because you're running low on energy. Avoid the slump with the following energy-boosting foods:

- **Freshly grated ginger:** A great stimulator to throw into smoothies, or whack it in a stir-fry.
- **Sweet potatoes:** A great carb to have; one serving brings total vitality to the day.
- **Nuts and seeds:** Walnuts contain the most omega-3s of all the nuts, and

are great for brain power.

- **Eggs:** Bursting with protein, these babies will keep you full and energised all day long.
- **Quinoa:** This grain is a great source of vegetarian protein. It packs a punch with a nice dose of folate, magnesium and phosphorus.

how to read food labels

- Choose foods with the fewest ingredients on the label.
- If it contains added sugar – bin it.
- Avoid any 'diet', 'low-fat' and '0% fat' labels.
- Only eat foods that contain words you understand – no crazy E numbers, please!
- Choose savoury foods that contain less than 6g of sugar per 100g.

should i go organic?

The way we farm and manufacture our food has changed. We import lots of our food from the other side of the world, and the manufacturers tend to load it with pesticides and preservatives.

However, I understand that buying organic often comes with a heftier price tag. I don't buy organic produce all the time, but certain fruit and veg are best bought organic, because more pesticides and chemicals are typically used in their production. I have therefore divided some common fruit and veg into the 'dirty dozen' and the 'clean fifteen'.

the dirty dozen: *buy these organic*	the clean fifteen: *no need to buy these organic*
apples	onions
celery	sweetcorn
peppers	pineapples
pears	avocado
strawberries	cabbage
grapes	peas
spinach	asparagus
lettuce	mangoes
cucumbers	aubergine
potatoes	kiwi
green beans	melon
kale	sweet potatoes
	grapefruit
	watermelon
	mushrooms

shop local

Choosing organic is the best option, but I think it's even more important to buy food that is grown locally. Much of the food we eat is grown thousands of miles away, meaning it takes longer to hit your dinner plate, during which time it loses nutrition and taste – not to mention polluting our beautiful planet to get there.

Locally bought food tastes fresh, can often work out cheaper and is good for the conscience.

how to eat local

- Do your weekly shop at a farmers' market.
- Get a local veg box delivery.
- Chose local produce over foreign.
- Eat seasonal produce; you can look up what's in season online.

super chef

Don't panic too much when it comes to cooking your food. The key is to use the right oils and not overdo the dish. Methods to avoid:

- Microwaving
- Over-boiling
- Burning (glycation) – burnt food can cause toxic build-up

- Deep frying

Instead, stick to:

- Boiling or steaming in a little water, keeping the crunch
- Grilling, roasting, baking or sautéing

Try cooking in coconut oil or butter; they both have high smoking points and do not denature in heat. Do not burn, though! Olive oil is OK for cooking at low temperatures or drizzling over at the end.

cook it slow and low

I have a total love affair with my slow cooker. It's the easiest way to get a good nourishing meal inside you. If you aren't much of a cook, it will be your best friend. All you have to do is pop a whole load of veg and meat in it, and – hey presto! – a restaurant-worthy dish appears. Often I'll leave mine on during the day while I'm out and about, and when I get home I'll open the door to a ready-made dinner.

They're cheap, they make meat melt off the bone . . . and it's only one pot to clean up at the end of a long day. Get into the habit of making a slow roast on a Sunday and eating the meat all week.

The best part about slow cooking is that you can use cheaper, less-popular cuts of meat like brisket, shoulder and neck. The slow cooker totally transforms these generally tougher cuts into delicacies. Also, cooking slow and low retains

more nutrients (those that are destroyed from the heat) for the body.

a final note from me

So you've got to the end of this endeavour, and you should feel very proud! Even if you only made one change, it is still a great leap in the right direction.

Get the Glow isn't just about losing weight or seeing better skin. It is that healthy, happy sheen that comes from within; it shines through in your habits, conviction and good wholesome nourishment.

You deserve this.

So walk with confidence, smile and GLOW!

I hope you enjoyed yourself; please stay in touch via my website, Facebook, Twitter and Instagram, and do keep me updated on your progress!

Lots of love,

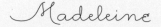

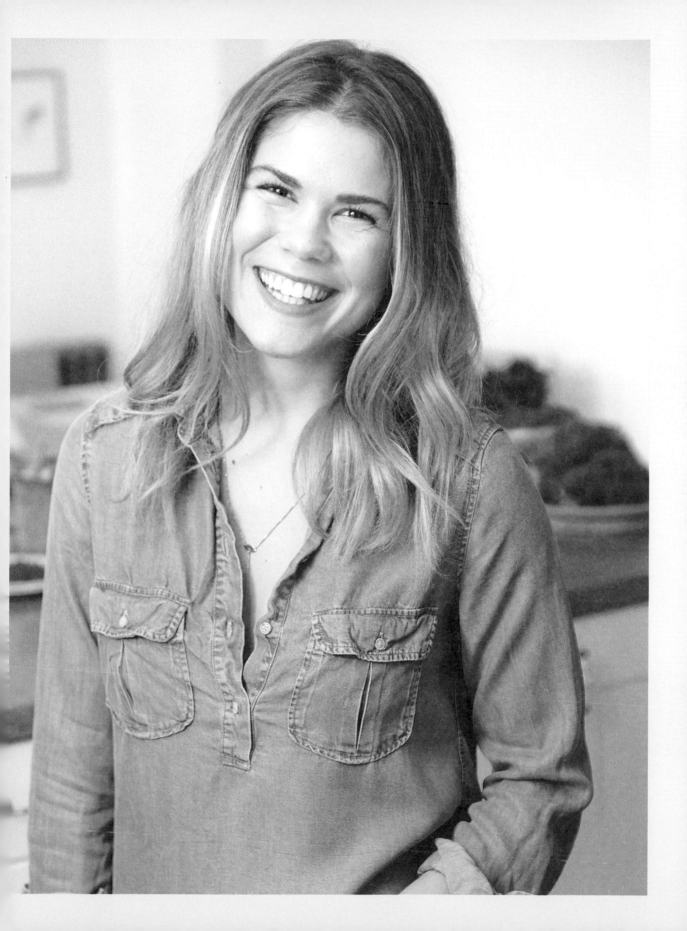

sample weekly meal plan

	monday	tuesday	wednesday
breakfast	simple overnight bircher (page 70)	scrambled eggs with pesto and avocado (page 72)	three-ingredient banana chia pudding (page 93)
lunch	smoked salmon and fattoush salad with avocado mash (page 149)	orange duck with charred chicory (page 166)	pan-fried ocean trout with a beetroot and pear salad (page 168)
snack	1 seedy energy bar (page 112)	1 spirulina ball (page 102)	rosemary spiced pecans (page 111)
dinner	orange duck with charred chicory (*make a portion for lunch the next day*) (page 166)	pan-fried ocean trout with a beetroot and pear salad (*make a portion for lunch the next day*) (page 168)	warm kale, chickpea and orange salad (*make a portion for lunch the next day*) (page 150)

thursday	friday	saturday	sunday
almond pancakes with grilled banana and walnuts (page 74)	raw berry buckwheat porridge (page 80)	poached egg, quinoa and beetroot bowl (page 88)	fried egg with bacon and roast vine tomatoes (page 90)
warm kale, chickpea and orange salad (page 150)	ginger steamed snapper parcel with cauliflower rice and chard (page 171)	mexican mince in lettuce wraps with fresh salsa (page 197)	butternut and coconut soup (*make a large batch for the week*) (page 122)
guacamole with beetroot and rosemary crackers (page 106)	1 protein ball (page 103)	1 raw chocolate ball (page 102)	1 red velvet cupcake with coconut whipped cream (page 220)
ginger steamed snapper parcel with cauliflower rice and chard (*make a portion for lunch the next day*) (page 171)	chickpea and lentil dhal with coconut cauliflower rice (page 194)	steak with parsnip chips (page 160)	slow-roast lamb shank (page 190)

recipes

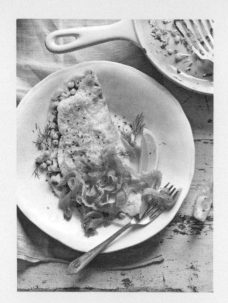

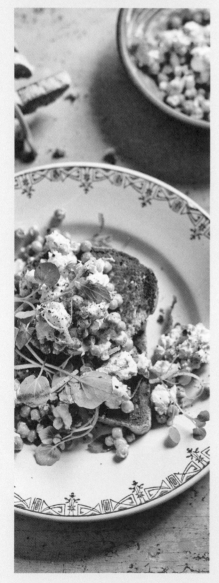

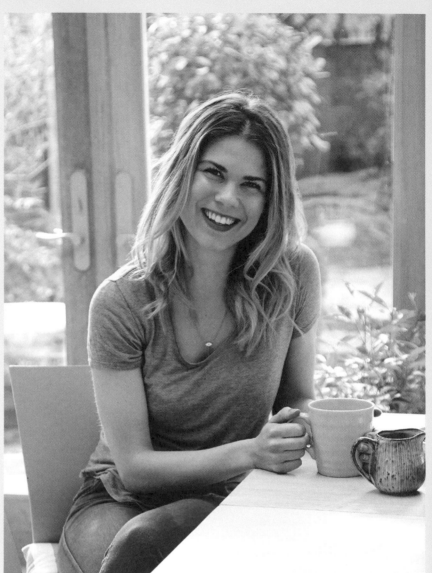

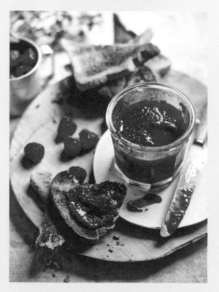

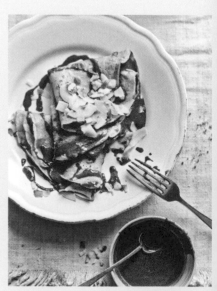

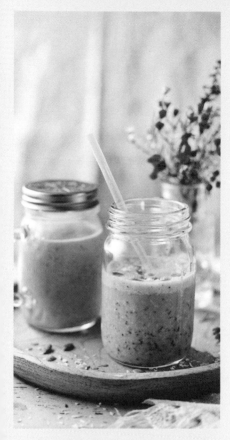

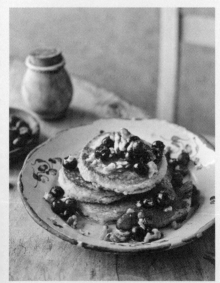

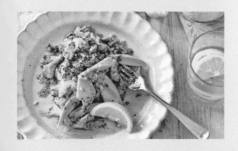

breakfast

simple overnight bircher

serves 2

150g gluten-free
  oats
300ml almond
  milk, plus extra
  for serving
pinch salt
1 tsp vanilla extract
2 tsp cinnamon
1 tsp coconut oil
50g pumpkin seeds
1 green apple
1 tsp honey
  (optional)
50g natural
  yoghurt

*This will keep in the
fridge for 1-2 days.*

I really got into bircher while living in Sydney. And I love this recipe: it's so simple – you just have to remember to prep it the night before to give the oats some soaking time. Swap the almond milk for other milks or fresh apple juice if you like. As the seasons change, pop in some seasonal fruit to give it another dimension. This is a great brekkie to make in a jam jar and bring to work; it might get a little mushed but the flavour will be just as fantastic.

The night before you want to eat the bircher, soak the oats with the milk, salt and vanilla extract in a bowl. Stir well, and put the bowl in the fridge overnight.

Pop the cinnamon, coconut oil and seeds in a frying pan over a low heat, and toast them for a few minutes. Leave to cool, then cover and set aside.

In the morning grab the oats from the fridge, grate the apple on top, stir in the honey if using, dollop on the yoghurt and sprinkle the cinnamon seeds over the top.

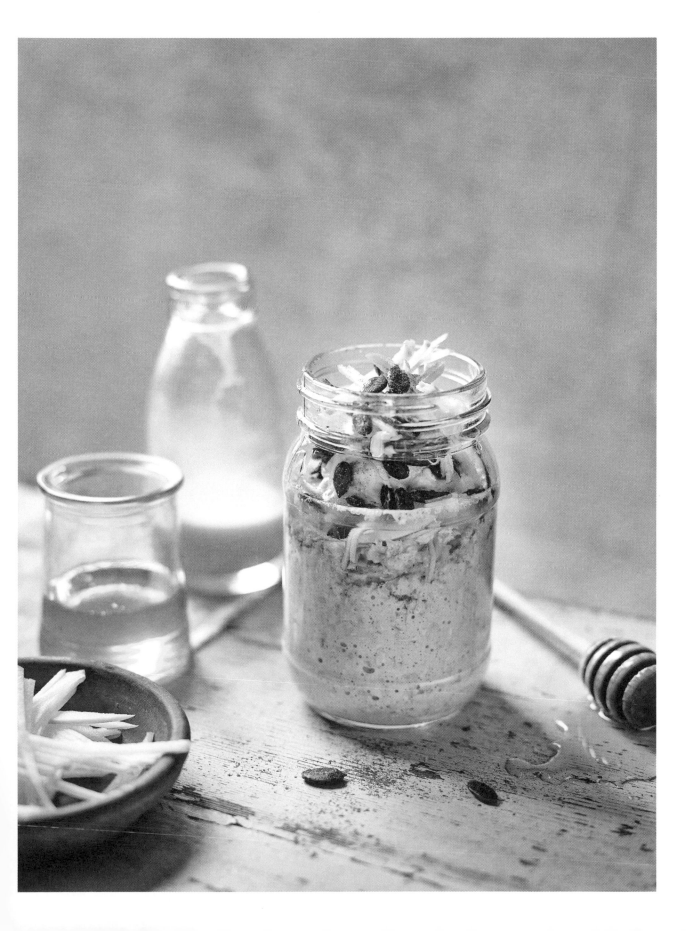

scrambled eggs with pesto and avocado

serves 1

3 eggs
50ml milk
1 tbsp coconut oil
  or butter

homemade pesto
1 lemon
1 clove garlic
40g walnuts, plus
  extra for topping
3 handfuls basil,
  finely chopped
6 tbsp olive oil

½ an avocado,
  sliced, to serve
salt and pepper

*Leftover pesto can keep
in the fridge for a week or
so. Slather it over salads
or more eggs.*

This homemade pesto is so fresh, and it takes to the eggs like a duck to water. Mix up the nuts – in this recipe I've used walnuts, but pine nuts work well too, or even cashews. When buying eggs, always get the best quality you can find: 'free range', 'pasture raised' or 'organic' are the key words you're looking for. Top-quality eggs mean more goodness for you.

Make the pesto. Zest and juice half of the lemon. Cut the other half into wedges and set aside. In a blender or food processor, blitz the garlic, walnuts, lemon zest and basil, slowly drizzling in the olive oil and the lemon juice as you do so.

Whisk the eggs and milk with a good grind of pepper and a pinch of salt. Heat the coconut oil or butter in a large frying pan over a medium-high heat for 1 minute. Turn down the heat slightly, then pour in the eggs and let the mixture sit for 15 seconds. With a wooden spoon or spatula start folding the outer ridge of the egg inwards to the centre. Add 2 tablespoons of the pesto, and fold the eggs and pesto together. Keep folding for a minute until the eggs are cooked through.

Serve with a couple of crushed walnuts, the lemon wedges, slices of avocado and some extra pesto if you like.

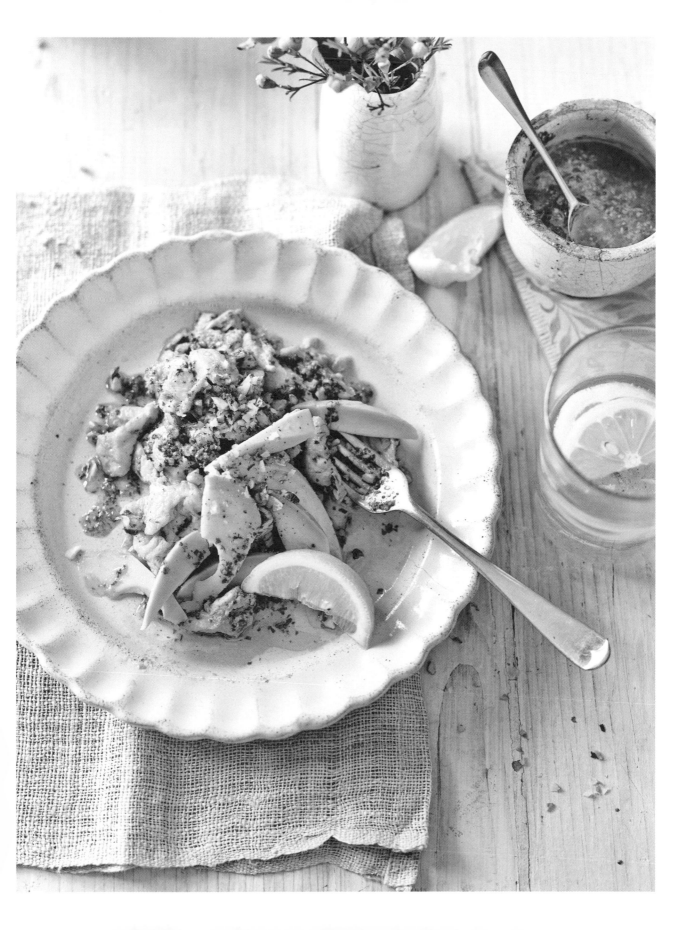

almond pancakes with grilled banana and walnuts

makes 9 pancakes

200g ground
  almonds
1 tsp baking
  powder
small pinch salt
2 eggs, lightly
  beaten
180ml almond milk
  (or other milk of
  your choice)
2 tbsp coconut oil
2 bananas
50g walnuts, finely
  chopped
1 tsp cinnamon,
  plus extra for
  dusting
blueberries,
  walnuts and
  honey, to serve

*The batter will keep in
the fridge for a few days,
so you can enjoy them a
few more times.*

Pancakes are the perfect weekend treat, and you can enjoy these ones guilt free. Your skin will be glowing thanks to the vitamin E-rich ground almond that forms the base of these beauties. The bananas provide a nice dose of potassium, so this treat is perfect post-workout.

In a bowl, mix the ground almonds, baking powder and salt. In another bowl, whisk the eggs with the milk. Slowly add the dry almond mixture to the egg mixture. Stir together vigorously, and leave in the fridge for at least 20 minutes, and up to 12 hours.

Heat the coconut oil in a frying pan over a medium heat for 1 minute. Remove the pancake batter from the fridge, and pour around 60ml batter into the pan. Cook until bronzed underneath (around 3 minutes), then flip and cook on the other side for another minute. Repeat with the rest of the pancakes. Stack them and keep them warm.

Slice the bananas in half lengthways. In a separate pan, heat 1 tablespoon coconut oil and the cinnamon over a medium heat for 1 minute. Place the banana halves in the pan, and cook for 2 minutes on each side until golden.

Serve the pancakes with the bananas, blueberries, walnuts, a drizzle of honey and a dusting of cinnamon.

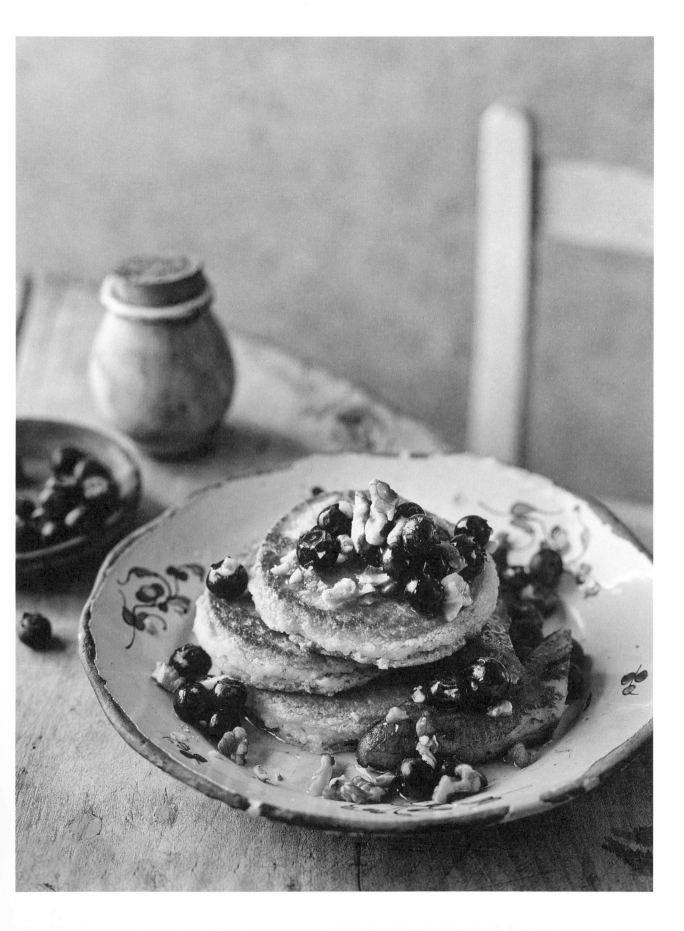

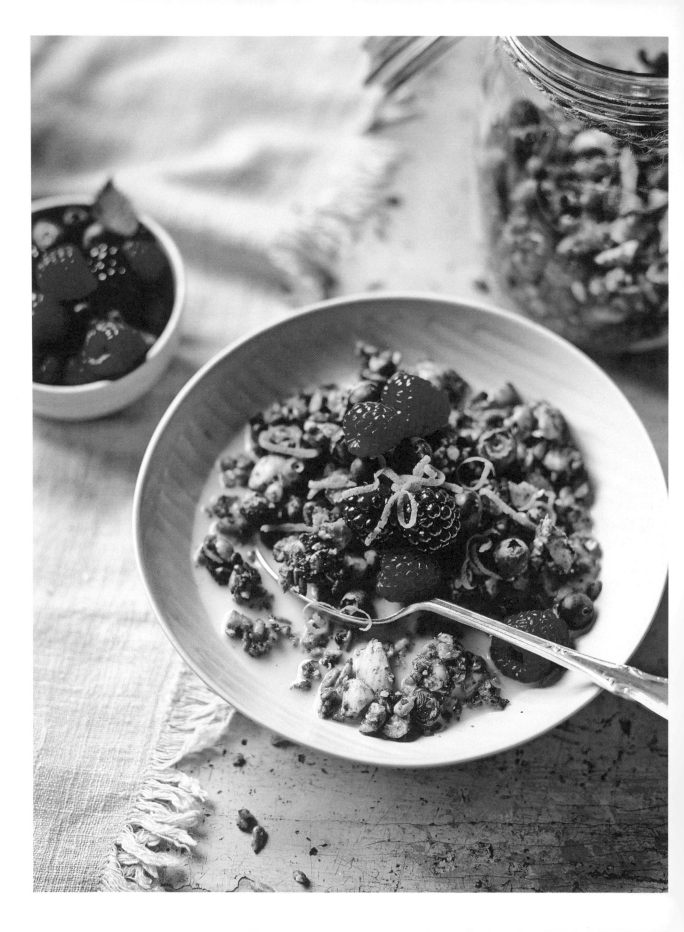

grain-free chocolate granola

This is a super brekkie for those who miss their cereal fix. You can make it on a Sunday to munch on throughout the week. There is no added sugar, but it relies on a slight sweetness from the banana and the nuts. Pour some delicious milk and berries over the top, and enjoy the crunch.

Preheat the oven to 180°C/350°F/Gas mark 4.

Whizz the nuts and seeds for just 20 seconds in a food processor – keep them crunchy.

Spread out the nuts on a baking sheet lined with baking paper. Meanwhile, blitz the banana, ginger, cinnamon, cacao and coconut oil in a food processor; blend to a paste. Pour this mixture onto the nuts, and combine thoroughly.

Cook in the oven for 20 minutes, until crisp. Remove and allow to cool, then top with the orange zest.

Serve bowlfuls with almond milk and some fresh berries.

serves 5

150g hazelnuts
150g almonds
150g walnuts
150g sunflower
  seeds
1 banana
1 tsp ground ginger
1 tsp cinnamon
2 tbsp raw cacao
1 tbsp coconut oil
zest of 1 orange
almond milk and
  berries, to serve

This will keep in an airtight container for a few weeks, so you can prep breakfasts in advance.

pea and dill omelette
with smoked salmon

Omelettes are great – you can mix up the contents and totally transform them. This one has a nice Nordic feel, thanks to the fresh dill and salmon. Adding lemon at the end brings everything together and is very alkalising for the body.

serves 1

1 tbsp butter or coconut oil
½ small white onion, finely chopped
1 small handful frozen peas
2 eggs
1 tsp chopped fresh dill
100g smoked salmon
½ lemon, cut into wedges
salt and pepper

Heat ½ tablespoon butter or coconut oil in an omelette pan for 1 minute, then add the onion and sauté for 5 minutes over a medium heat. Add the peas and stir for another minute. Tip the cooked veg onto a plate and put to one side.

Whisk the eggs in a bowl, and heat the remaining ½ tablespoon butter or coconut oil in the pan over a medium heat for 1 minute. Pour in the egg mixture, let it cover the sides of the pan, and after 30 seconds, use a wooden spoon to gently push the sides of the eggs towards the centre, allowing the uncooked egg mix to move into the gaps. Throw in the dill, a pinch of salt and the pea and onion mix so they are on top of the eggs. Fold the omelette in half and allow it to cook for another 30 seconds, then serve with smoked salmon, freshly ground pepper and lemon wedges.

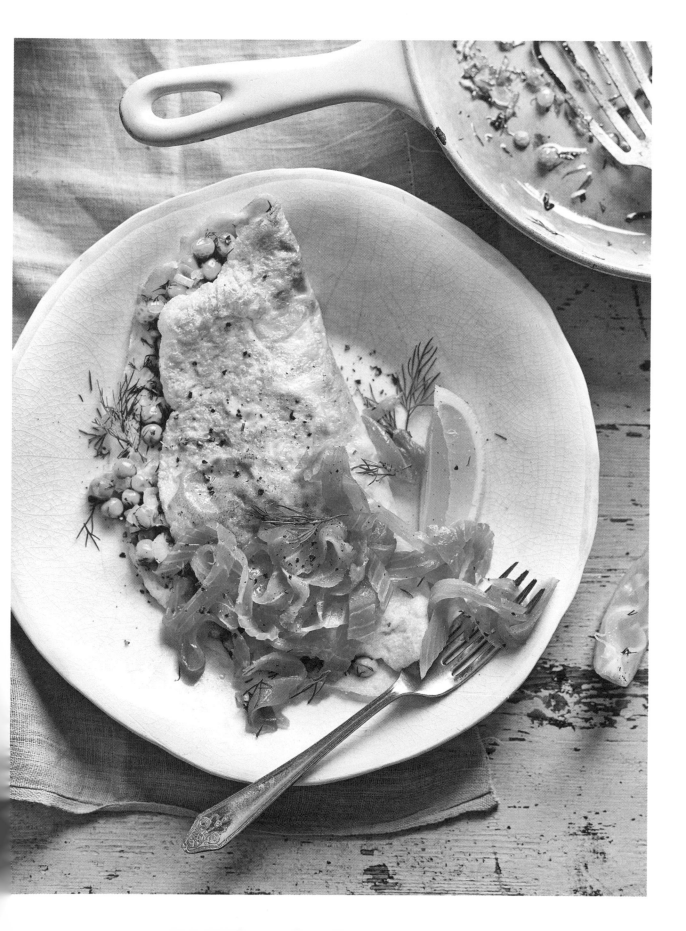

raw berry buckwheat porridge

This breakfast is such a delight. I love the soft texture, which complements the bursting flavours from the zest and cinnamon. This is another great brekkie that you can take with you to work or make in advance. It's raw, so it retains all the goodness from each nutrient-dense food I have included. Enjoy!

serves 2
100g buckwheat
100g cashew nuts
50g strawberries, hulled and sliced
zest and juice of 1 orange
½ tsp vanilla extract
1 tsp cinnamon
1 tbsp honey

extra toppings
pumpkin seeds (or other seeds of your choice)
desiccated coconut
cinnamon
mixed berries

The night before you want to eat the porridge, soak the buckwheat and the cashew nuts in separate bowls with enough water to cover.

In the morning, drain the water from the buckwheat and nuts and blend them in a food processor with the rest of the ingredients.

Serve with some extra berries, your choice of seeds, coconut and a dusting of cinnamon.

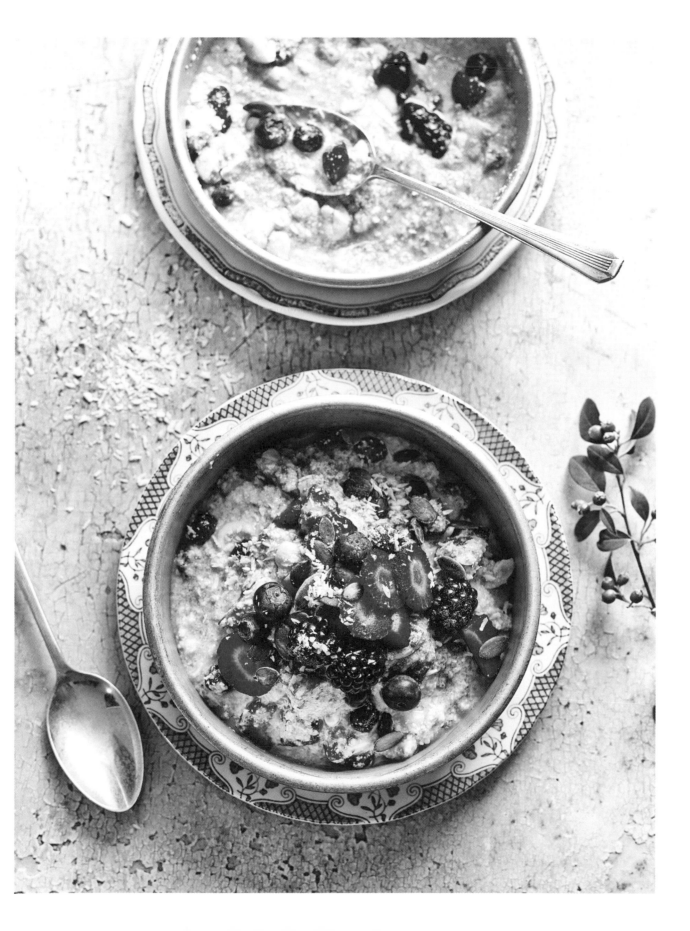

goat's cheese, pea and mint smash

Inspired by breakfast spots in Sydney, this savoury number takes minutes to make – and I know it won't last long on the plate. Goat's cheese is much easier to digest than other cheeses, and is abundant in vitamins D, K and A. It goes so well with the fresh mint and peas; this melt-in-the-mouth dish will send you to another world.

serves 2

zest and juice of 1 lemon
150g goat's cheese
1 tbsp chopped fresh mint
100g petits pois frozen
2 slices toasted gluten-free bread,
  homemade Quinoa Bread (see page 96)
  or rye bread
20g watercress
salt and pepper

Mix the lemon zest and juice with the goat's cheese, mint, petits pois, a pinch of salt and freshly ground pepper. Let this sit for a few minutes to allow the petits pois to defrost the flavours to infuse, then slather on some toast and serve with the watercress.

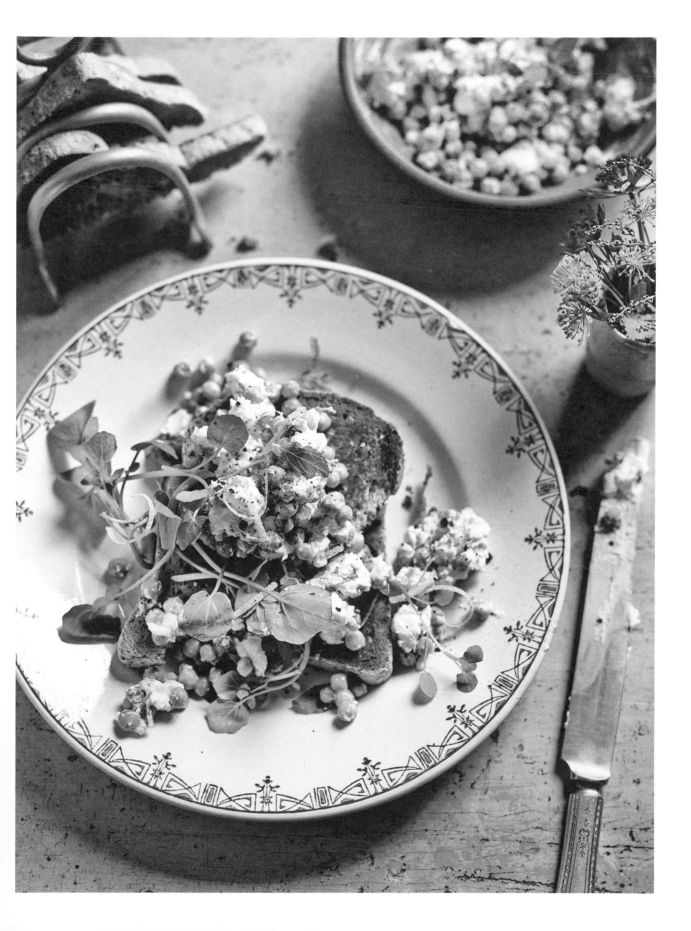

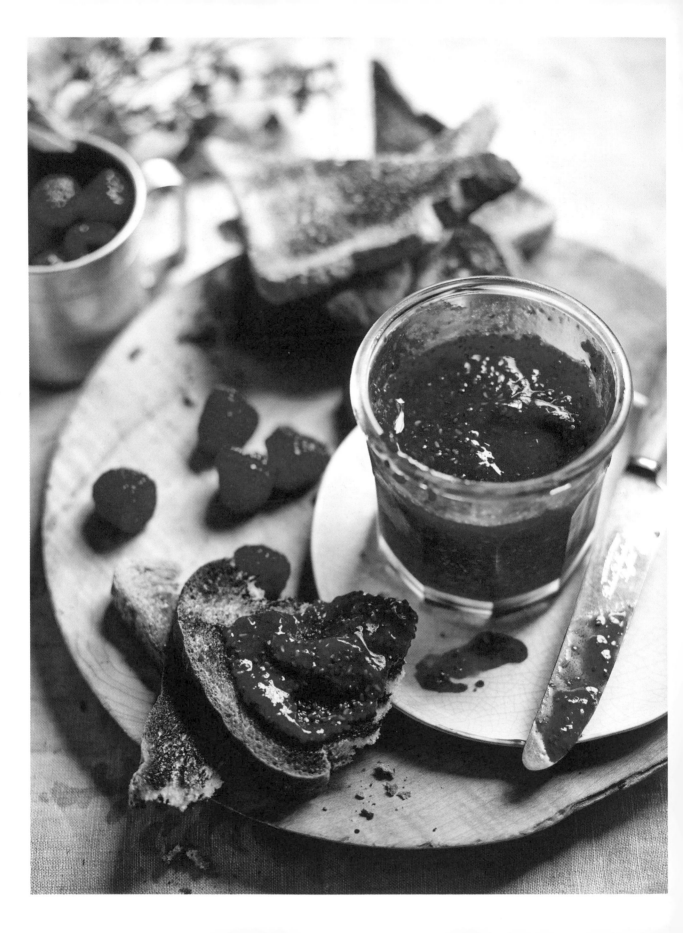

chia raspberry jam

There is nothing quite like homemade jam, especially one that is good for you. The chia seeds act as a binding agent, bringing this spread together and giving it that jammy quality. The result is sweet, gooey goodness.

makes about 200g
200g raspberries
1 tbsp honey
½ tsp vanilla extract
2½ tbsp chia seeds

Put the raspberries, honey and vanilla in a blender or food processor, and blend until smooth. Pour into a bowl, then stir in the chia seeds and mix vigorously by hand.

Pop the mixture in a jar and chill in the fridge for 15 minutes to allow it to set. Serve smeared on my Quinoa Bread (page 96), gluten-free or rye bread.

The jam keeps for 4 days in the fridge.

chocolate hazelnut crêpes

serves 2–3 (makes around 6 crêpes)

chocolate hazelnut
  spread
300g skinless
  hazelnuts
2 tbsp coconut oil
4 tbsp raw cacao
pinch salt
75g coconut sugar

crêpes
4 eggs
225ml almond milk
  (or other milk of
  your choice)
125g buckwheat
  flour
pinch salt
3 tbsp toasted
  coconut flakes,
  to serve

*The batter will keep in
the fridge for a few days,
so you can enjoy these
a few more times. The
finished 'nutella' keeps in
the fridge for 1 week.*

Crêpes are among my favourite breakfasts, and this recipe reminds me of Paris. They are a winner with my boyfriend, and will get any man thinking that healthy eating is easy. The chocolate hazelnut spread or 'nutella' is so gooey, and the coconut sugar gives it a nice caramel taste. You will definitely find me dipping my finger into the pot late at night.

Preheat the oven to 150°C/300°F/Gas mark 2.

To make the 'nutella', spread the hazelnuts out in a roasting tin, and roast for 15 minutes; watch these babies carefully so they don't burn. Grind them in a food processor with 1 tablespoon coconut oil for 5 minutes. Add the raw cacao, a pinch of salt and the coconut sugar. Blend for another 5–10 minutes until smooth.

To make the crêpes, whisk the eggs and milk in a large bowl, then slowly sift in the flour with the final pinch of salt.

Heat 1 tablespoon coconut oil in a frying pan over a medium heat, and swirl the oil around to cover the base of the pan.

Pour about 50ml of the batter into the pan, making sure the mixture is evenly distributed. When the edges are set and they start to curl up (after about 1 minute) flip the crêpe over and dollop a few tablespoons of 'nutella' into the middle of the crêpe. Smear it around, but leave at least a couple of centimetres around the edges of the crêpe. Cook for 30 seconds, then fold in half.

Repeat the process to use up the mixture for the rest of the crêpes. Serve with a sprinkle of toasted coconut flakes.

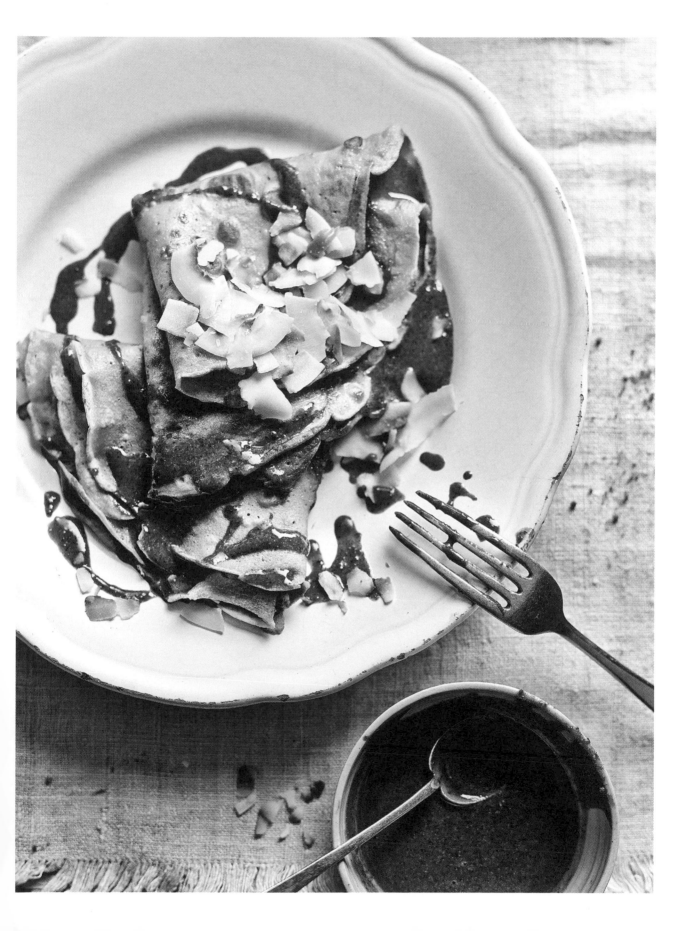

poached egg, quinoa and beetroot bowl

Poaching eggs is a great way to enjoy them – I love mine with the soft, runny yolk oozing all over the plate. And raw beetroot is amazing; grating it is such a simple way of getting it into your diet. This breakfast is pure protein power, with a nice dose coming from both the eggs and the quinoa. There will be nothing stopping you after this.

serves 1

75g quinoa, rinsed
2 pinches salt
1 tsp cider vinegar
2 eggs
1 small beetroot, grated
3 tbsp olive oil
1 tbsp finely chopped fresh chives

chia seeds and pumpkin seeds, to sprinkle (optional)

Put the quinoa in a saucepan with 125ml water and a pinch of salt. Bring it to the boil, then turn the heat down and let it gently simmer for 12–15 minutes, or until all the water has been absorbed.

Boil around 200ml water in a small saucepan (ensure the water is at least 2.5cm deep). Add the cider vinegar and a pinch of salt, then keep at a high simmer. Crack the eggs individually into small ramekins. Drop each egg into the pan of simmering water and poach for 2–3 minutes, then remove the eggs with a slotted spoon.

Mix the quinoa with the grated beetroot, olive oil and chives, then top with the poached eggs and sprinkle over some chia seeds and pumpkin seeds if you would like an extra dose of omega-3 goodness.

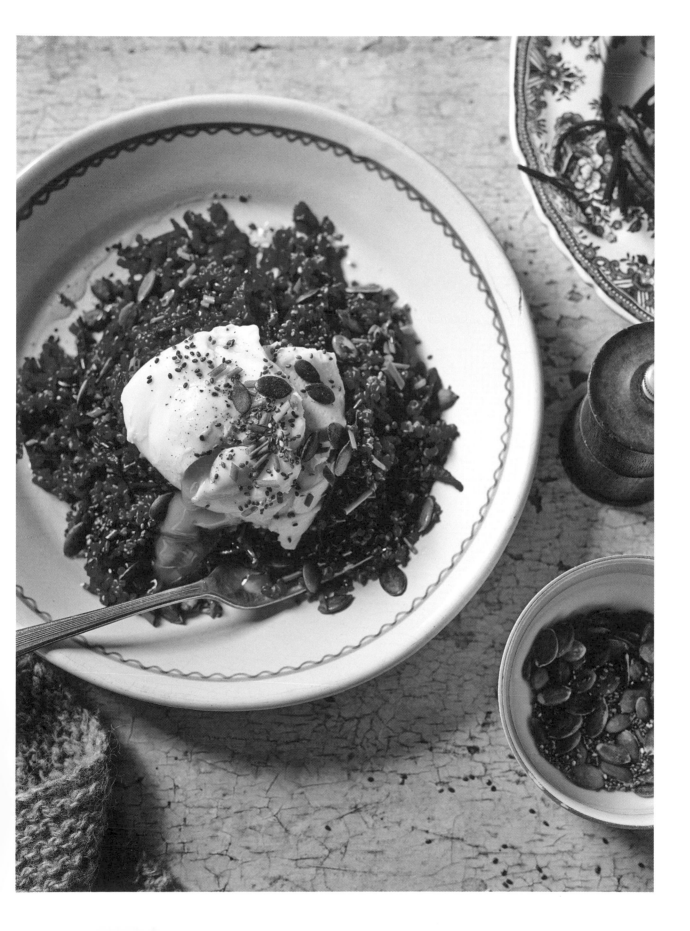

fried egg with bacon and roast vine tomatoes

People have the misconception that fried eggs are unhealthy. Well yes, if you fry them in vegetable oil – but these babies come cooked in the goodness of coconut oil. The roast tomatoes burst out of their skins, and team so well with the saltiness of the bacon and the luscious egg yolk.

serves 1

1 vine cherry tomatoes
2 tbsp coconut oil or butter, melted
1 tsp dried oregano
2 eggs
2 bacon rashers
salt and pepper

Preheat the oven to 180°C/350°F/Gas mark 4. Put the tomatoes (still on the vine) in a roasting tin, and brush them with 1 tablespoon coconut oil or butter, and the oregano. Roast in the oven for 12–15 minutes.

Heat the remaining 1 tablespoon coconut oil or butter in a frying pan over a high heat for 1 minute. Crack the eggs in, then put a lid on the pan. Cook for 1–2 minutes depending on whether you like them runny or well done.

In a griddle pan, cook the bacon to your liking. Serve everything together with a good pinch of salt and a grind of pepper.

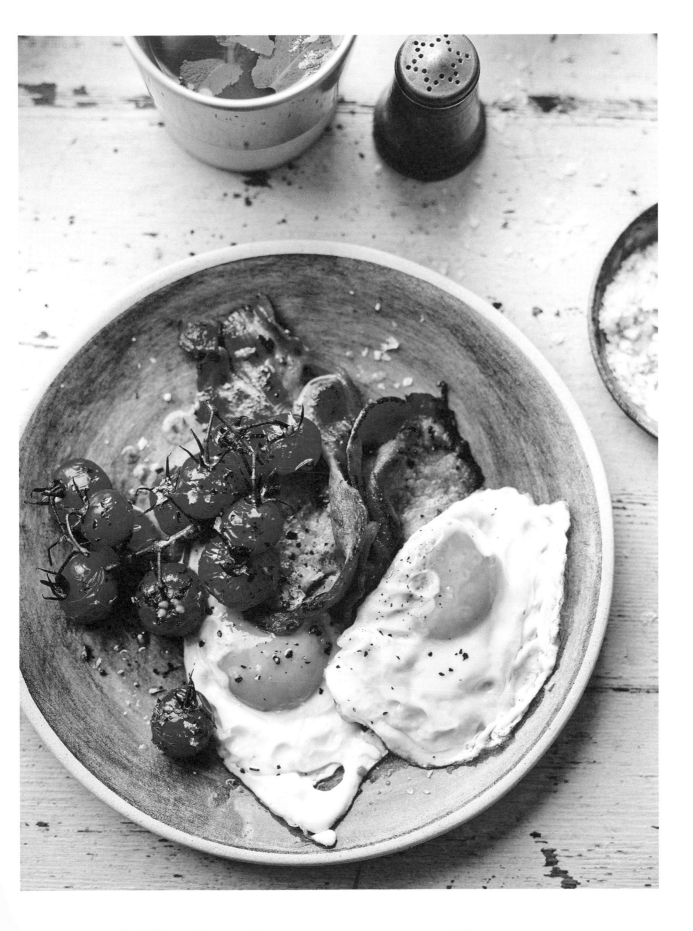

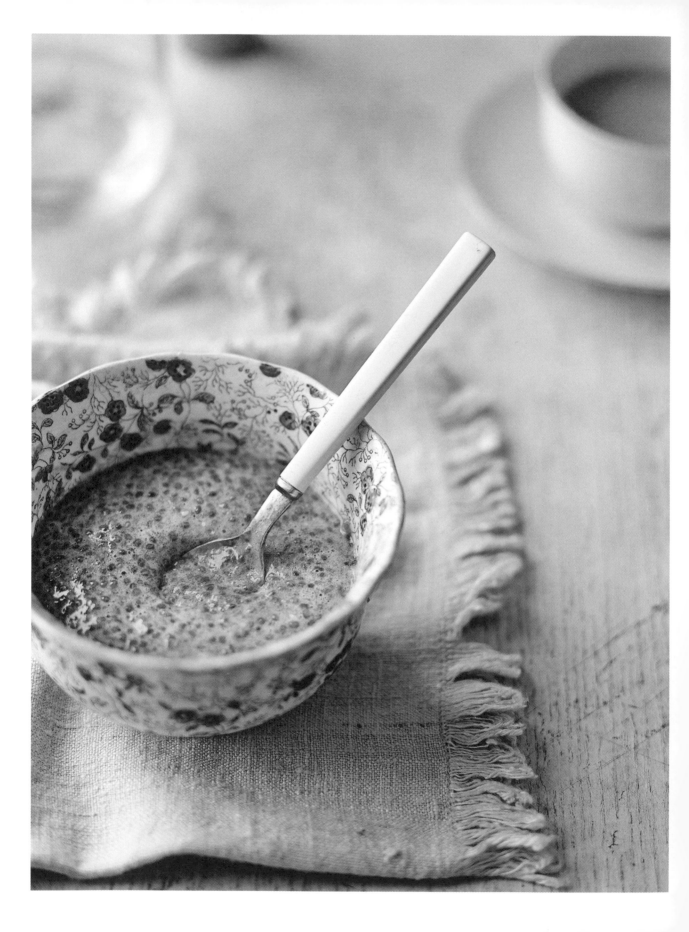

three-ingredient banana chia pudding

Unbelievably simple, yet wonderfully refined. With just three ingredients, this omega-3-loaded powerhouse will get your skin glowing. Chia seeds are hydrophilic, meaning that they absorb their weight in water, so this dish will hydrate your skin amazingly. Enjoy it as a light breakfast, pudding or as a quick snack on the go.

serves 1
1 very ripe banana, roughly chopped
100ml coconut milk
2 tbsp chia seeds

Put the banana and the coconut milk into a blender, and blitz for 2 minutes. Pour the mixture into a container, then stir in the chia seeds. Stir every few minutes for 10 minutes, then leave it in the fridge until set.

folded eggs with asparagus and lemon salsa

serves 1

70g asparagus
2 eggs
30ml almond milk,
 or other milk of
 your choice
1 tbsp coconut oil
 or butter

lemon salsa
zest and juice of
 1 lemon
1 tbsp finely
 chopped fresh
 mint
¼ red onion, finely
 chopped
1 tbsp olive oil
salt and pepper

Since discovering the technique of folding eggs I have never looked back; it creates the most wonderful velvety texture. The more love you give your eggs, the more love they give back. They're like men! Always go for pasture-raised eggs with a rich yolk – this is where all the vital minerals and nutrients are held. Balanced with the asparagus and lemon salsa, this spring breakfast will help you start your day fully fresh and energised.

Cut the ends off the asparagus, then put them in a small saucepan with a little boiling water and the tips pointing up. Steam for 5 minutes, or until cooked through.

To make the salsa, put the lemon zest and juice into a bowl, then add the mint, onion and 1 tablespoon olive oil. Grind in some pepper and salt and pour over the cooked asparagus.

In a bowl, whisk the eggs and milk with a good grind of pepper and a pinch of salt. Heat the coconut oil or butter in a frying pan over a medium-high heat for 2 minutes. Turn down the heat slightly and pour in the egg mixture. Let this sit for 15 seconds then, with a wooden spoon or spatula, start folding the outer ridge of the egg inwards to the centre, letting the uncooked egg flow into the gaps. Repeat this around the pan so that the egg cooks in folds rather than a messy scramble. Continue folding for another minute until the egg is cooked through, and serve with the salsa.

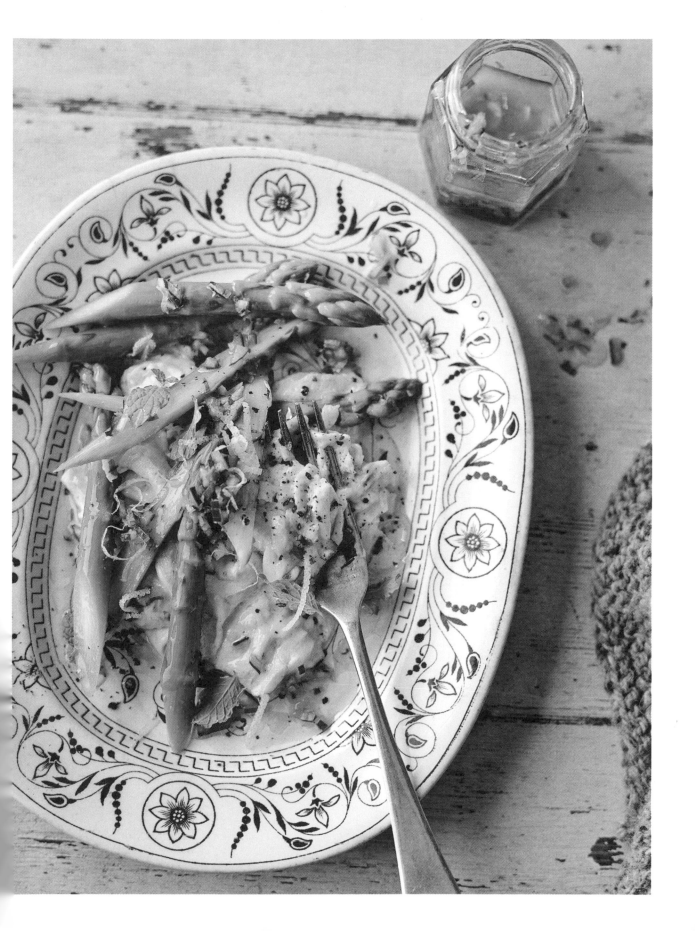

quinoa bread

It's so nice to have a gluten-free option for bread. This dense malt loaf is packed with protein from the quinoa, and the pecan nuts provide a healthy dose of selenium and vitamin E to make your skin glow.

serves 6

300g quinoa, oat or buckwheat flakes
200g pecan nuts
150g sunflower seeds, plus 10g for topping
¾ tbsp sea salt
1 tbsp chia seeds
500ml water
3 tbsp coconut oil, melted, plus extra for greasing

Mix all the dry ingredients together in a bowl, then slowly add the water and stir in the coconut oil. Leave to soak for 3-6 hours.

Preheat the oven to 180°C/350°F/Gas mark 4.

Grease a 900g loaf tin with coconut oil, then put the dough into the tin and put it in the oven. Bake for 40 minutes, then take the bread out of the tin and allow it to cook for another 40 minutes on a baking sheet in the oven so it gets cooked all over.

Let the bread cool on a cooling rack, then slice it up and enjoy.

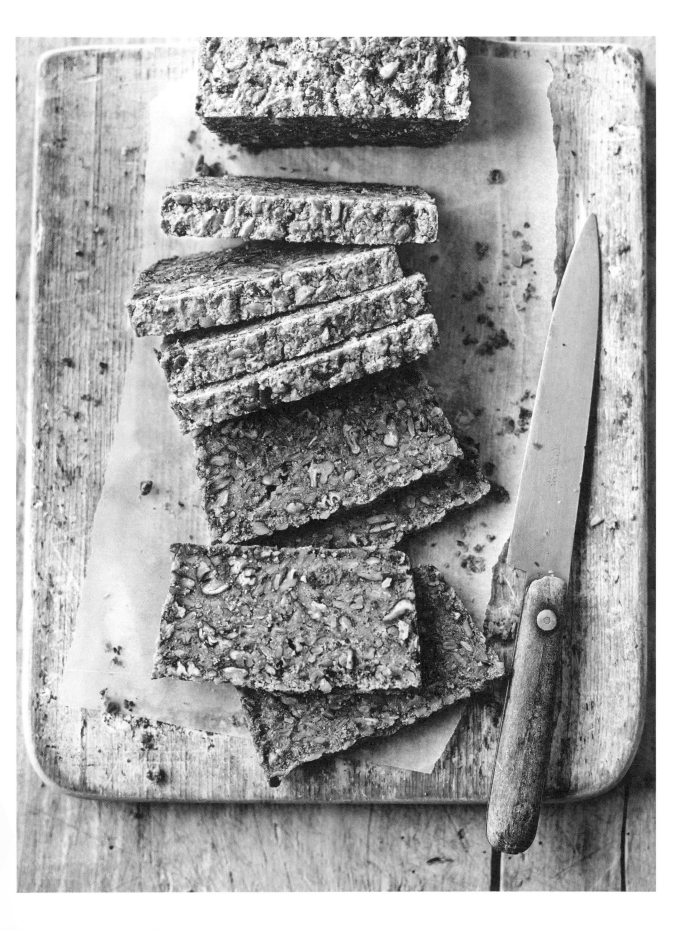

glowing green breakfast smoothie

serves 1

1 ripe avocado
250ml nut milk, or
   other milk of your
   choice
juice of 1 lime
¼ cucumber
20g cashew nuts

This smoothie gives you all the healthy benefits of avocado, with its skin-glowing vitamin E. The clean, zingy lime paired with the creaminess of nut milk really makes this smoothie come alive.

Blend all the ingredients together, and enjoy.
This can be made the night before, and lasts for a day in the fridge.

breakfast smoothie bowl

serves 1

1 frozen banana
   (peeled and
   frozen the night
   before)
50g frozen
   blueberries
250ml nut milk,
   rice milk, coconut
   milk or coconut
   water
1 tsp vanilla extract
   or powder
1 tbsp each of
   chia seeds,
   pumpkin seeds
   and desiccated
   coconut, for
   topping

I love this recipe's versatility, with it being half smoothie, half goodness bowl! Freezing a banana gives you a wonderful ice cream texture and flavour, without the guilt. The exotic blend of blueberries and banana is beautifully balanced with the natural sweetness of vanilla.

Blend together the banana, blueberries, milk or coconut water and vanilla, then put them in a bowl and top with the seeds and coconut. Eat immediately.

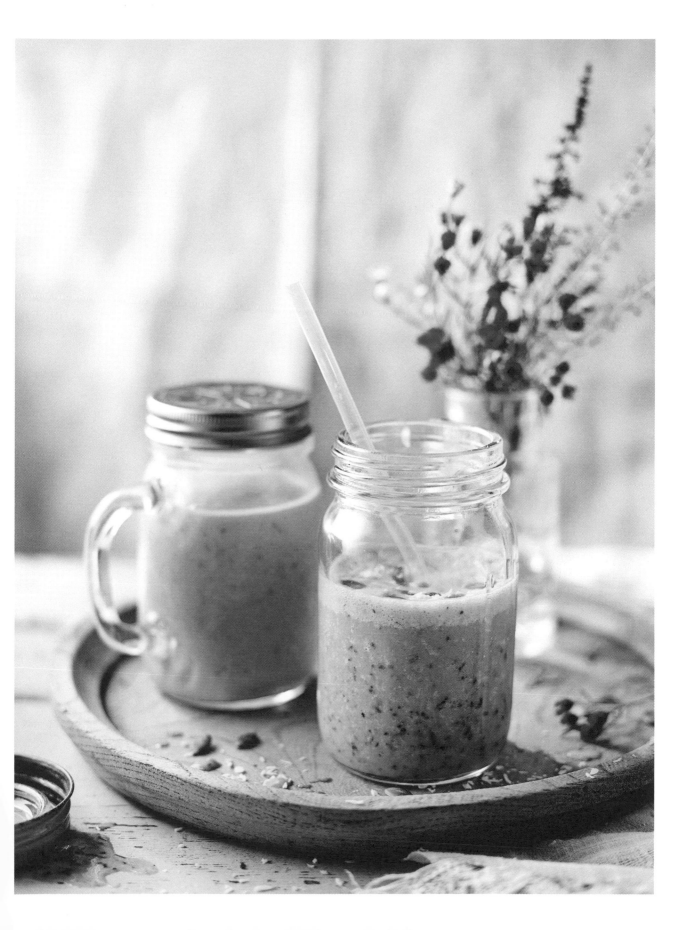

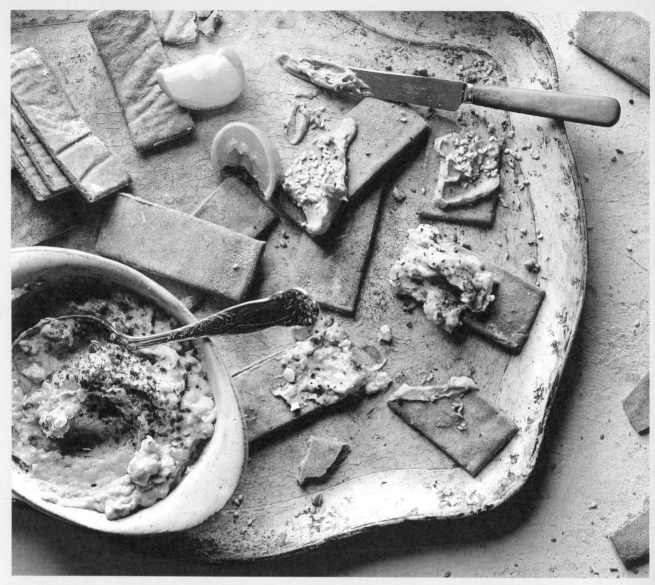

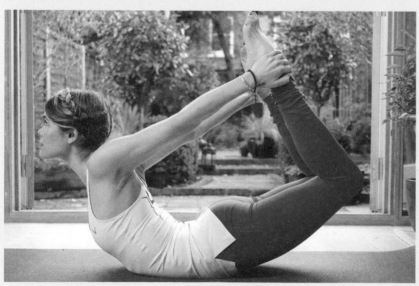

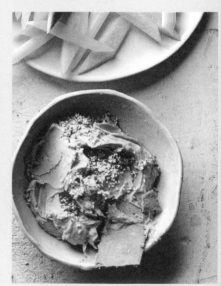

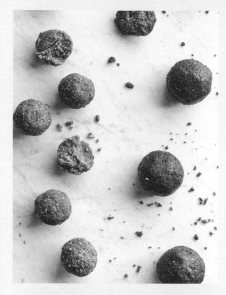

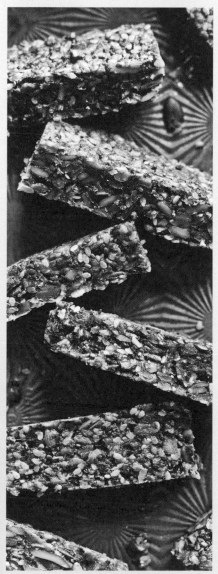

snacks

raw superfood balls

spirulina balls

makes 10–12 balls

100g cashew nuts
150g pumpkin
    seeds
tiny pinch salt
1 tsp cinnamon
1 tsp spirulina
200g Medjool dates
2 tbsp coconut oil
zest of 1 small
    orange

Spirulina is a total superfood, loaded with beta-carotene, iron, calcium, magnesium, vitamin B complex and chlorophyll … yes, the list is almost endless. It's quite powerful stuff, so here I've mixed it with dates, cinnamon and coconut to make it super-enjoyable.

Blend the nuts and seeds in a food processor for a minute, then add the rest of the ingredients, blend to allow everything to combine, roll the mixture into balls and pop them in the fridge. Leave them to set for an hour, then enjoy.

These will keep in the fridge for 2 weeks.

raw chocolate balls

makes 10–12 balls

100g hazelnuts
100g desiccated
    coconut
100g fresh dates
50g raw cacao
3 tbsp coconut oil
tiny pinch salt

These are a classic – whizz them up on a Sunday and snack happily all week long. I like to add a little salt to bring out the chocolaty taste and the desiccated coconut gives a tropical feel to these mind-blowing snacks.

Blend the nuts in a food processor for 1 minute, then add the rest of the ingredients and blend for 3–4 minutes until they are thoroughly mixed. Roll the mixture into balls and pop them in the freezer for 20 minutes, then transfer to the fridge.

These will keep in the fridge for 2 weeks.

post-workout balls

It is essential to eat after a workout. The addition of protein powder helps the muscles recover quickly – these balls will get you back to the gym the next day, no problem.

Put everything into a food processor, and blend for 3–4 minutes until thoroughly mixed. Roll the mixture into balls and pop them in the freezer for 20 minutes, then transfer to the fridge.

These will keep in the fridge for 2 weeks.

makes 8–10 balls

50g peanut butter
100g desiccated coconut
100g dates, stoned and roughly chopped
2 tbsp raw protein powder
1 tsp cinnamon
1 tsp vanilla powder or extract

protein balls

These power balls will give your beautiful body an energy boost. Loaded with maca – a superfood that boosts vitality as well as libido – and sweetened with a touch of antioxidant-rich honey, these balls are the perfect snack to get you up and going.

In the food processor, blend the oats and almonds for 1–2 minutes, then add the cacao, maca and salt. Blend for 1 minute, then add the honey, almond butter and coconut oil. Blend, then roll the mixture into balls and put them in the fridge to set for a few hours.

These will keep in the fridge for 2 weeks.

makes 12–14 balls

100g oats
150g almonds
50g raw cacao
1 tbsp maca powder
pinch of salt
3 tbsp honey
100g almond butter
2 tbsp coconut oil

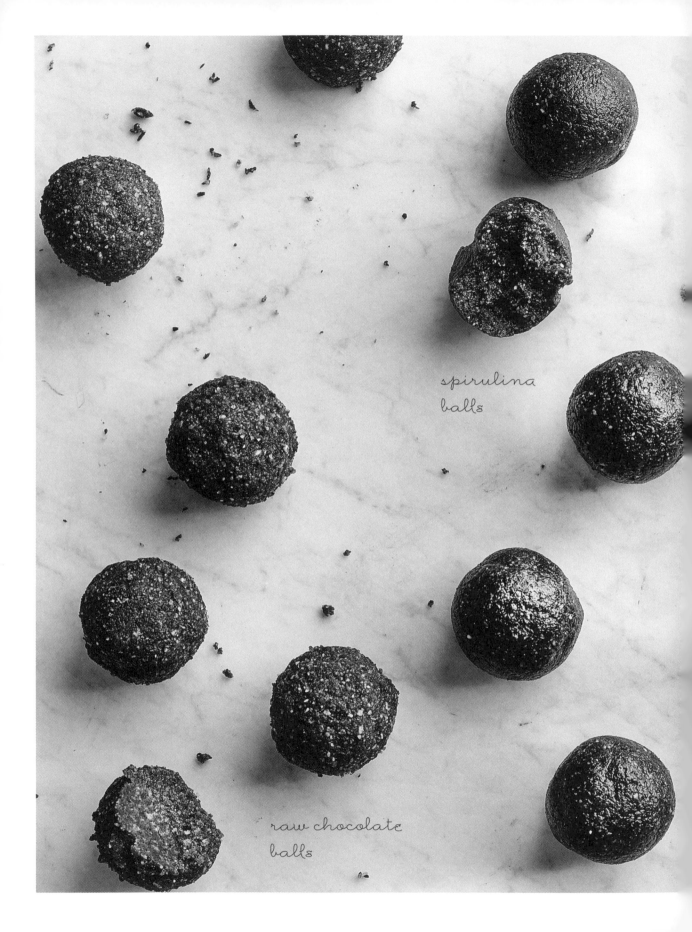

spirulina
balls

raw chocolate
balls

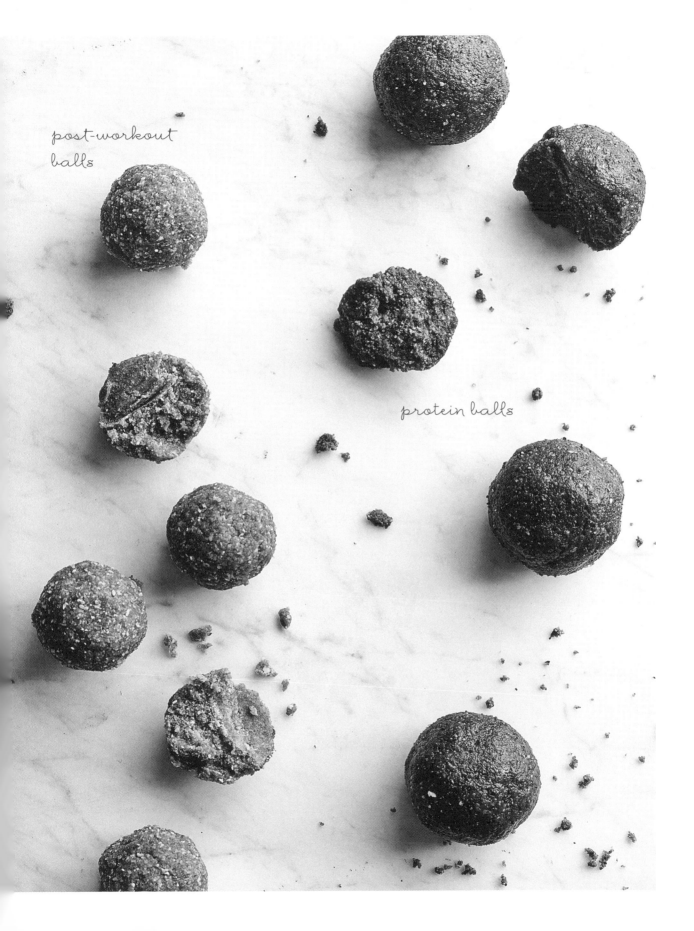

post-workout
balls

protein balls

guacamole with beetroot and rosemary crackers

I try and get avocado into everything. This guac (pictured overleaf) has a nice kick to it from the cayenne and chilli, and the lime adds a Mexican vibe. Spread this over everything: it's great on toast in the morning, too. As for the crackers, I struggle to find good-quality crackers that aren't laden with wheat and sugar – these are simple to make, and oh-so-tasty. Dip them in everything!

serves 4

2 avocados
2 limes
good pinch sea salt
1 tsp chilli flakes
pinch cayenne pepper, to taste
1 tbsp extra virgin olive oil

Slice open the avocados and scoop out the flesh. Put the rest of the ingredients apart from the extra virgin olive oil into a bowl, and gently mash with a fork.

Drizzle over the extra virgin olive oil, and serve sprinkled with extra cayenne if you like.

The guacamole keeps for 2 days in the fridge.

rosemary crackers

makes around 30 crackers

1 small beetroot
150g rice flour, buckwheat flour or ground almonds
1 tbsp dried rosemary
1 tsp salt
1 tsp freshly ground black pepper
2 free-range eggs
3 tbsp coconut oil or butter, melted and cooled

Preheat the oven to 180°C/350°F/Gas mark 4. Peel and grate the beetroot and squeeze 1 tablespoon of juice from the gratings into a bowl.

Put the flour or ground almonds, beetroot juice, rosemary, salt and pepper into a bowl, and mix together.

Put the eggs and coconut oil or butter in a separate bowl with the melted and cooled oil or butter, and whisk them together. Pour this into the dry mixture, and massage until it forms a dough. If it is too dry, add a little water.

Grab some baking paper and use it to line a large, flat baking sheet, then cut out another strip of baking paper the same size. Place the dough between the two sheets of baking paper and, with a rolling pin, roll it out in a 30cm square.

Cut the dough into 24 rectangular crackers with a sharp knife. Use the knife to wedge thin gaps between the crackers so they cook separately.

Bake for 15 minutes until golden and crispy. Flip them halfway through to ensure even cooking.

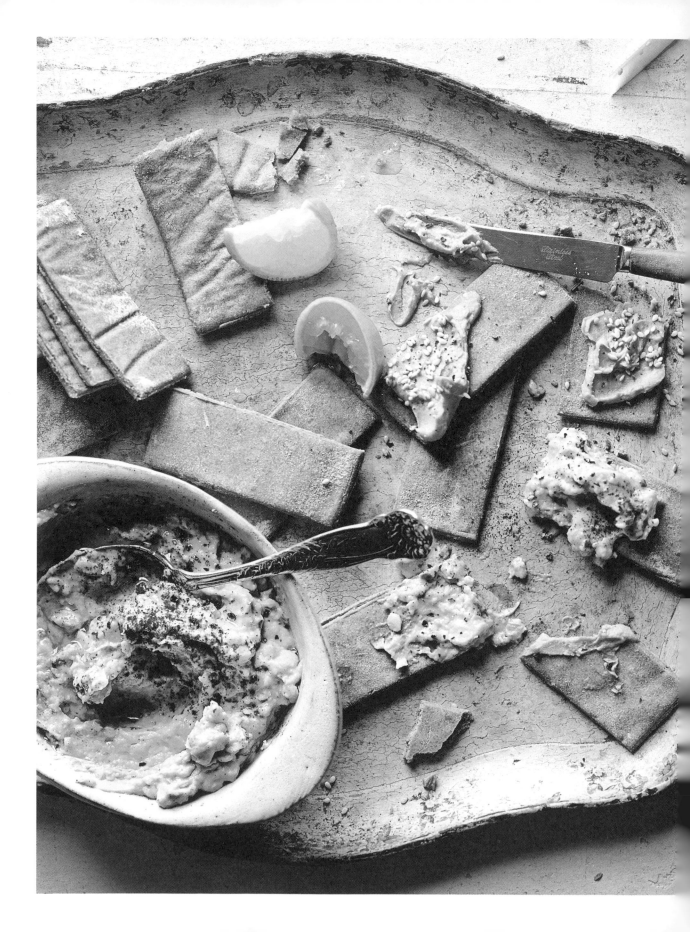

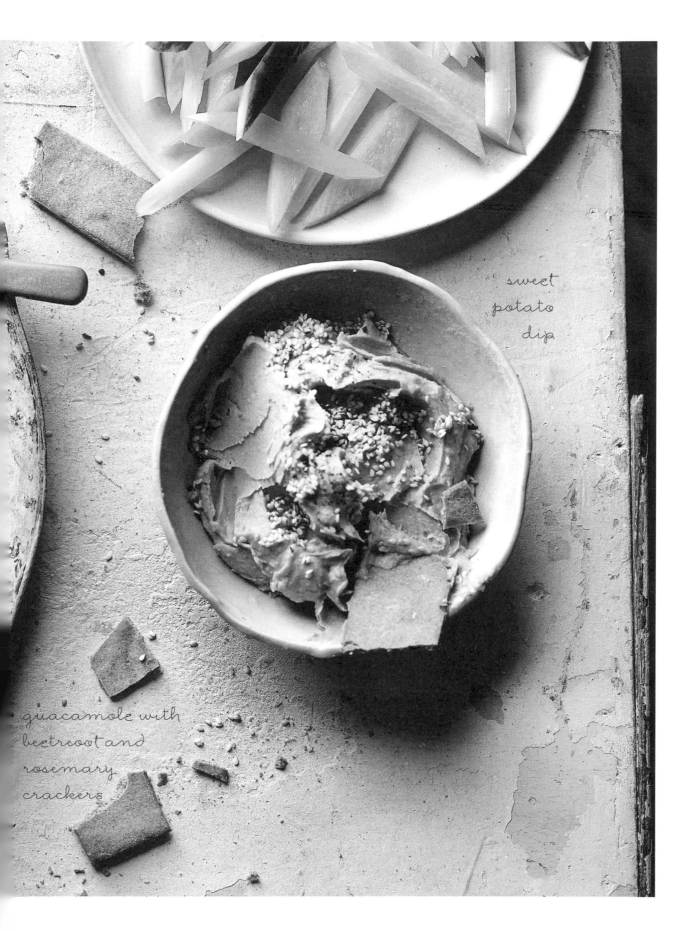

sweet
potato
dip

guacamole with
beetroot and
rosemary
crackers

sweet potato dip

This dip is insane. Creamy and spicy and full of goodness. Slather it over everything – poached eggs, crackers … the list is endless.

makes about 250g
250g sweet potato, peeled and cut into 2.5cm pieces
2 tsp ground ginger
4 tsp coconut cream
2 tbsp tahini
2 tsp gluten-free tamari, soy sauce or Liquid Aminos
2 tbsp sesame seeds
salt and pepper

Boil the sweet potato for 20 minutes, or until soft, in around 100ml water with a pinch of salt. Drain in a colander and reserve the liquid.

In a food processor blend the sweet potato, ginger, coconut cream, tahini and tamari, soy sauce or Liquid Aminos. Blend until smooth, and add a little of the sweet potato cooking water to thin it out if you want.

Toast the sesame seeds in a dry frying pan for 1 minute, stirring constantly so they don't burn. Put the sweet potato mixture in a bowl, and top with the toasted sesame seeds and some ground pepper. Leave to cool, then refrigerate.

Serve chilled, with vegetable crudités (pictured on page 109).

rosemary spiced pecans

These are the perfect snack, spiced with fresh rosemary and smoked paprika. Serve them on their own as a pre-dinner party snack, or throw them over soups and salads – these nuts seems to go with everything.

makes about 200g

1 tbsp coconut oil
200g pecan nuts
1 tsp salt
2 tbsp finely chopped fresh rosemary
1 tsp smoked paprika

Preheat the oven to 160°C/325°F/Gas mark 3.

Melt the coconut oil over a low heat. Toss all the other ingredients into a bowl and pour the oil over the top, then massage the spices into the oily pecan nuts.

Spread the nuts out onto a roasting tray and pop into the oven for 25 minutes. Halfway through the cooking time give the nuts a stir so that they cook evenly. Cool before eating.

seedy energy bars

My energy bars are a nut-free snack that will boost your energy levels and keep you fuller for longer. They contain an array of textures and flavours, healthy seeds marrying with the calcium-loaded tahini. No more afternoon tiredness.

makes 12 bars

1 ripe banana
2 tbsp coconut oil, plus extra for greasing
4 tbsp tahini
pinch salt
1 tsp cinnamon
100g pumpkin seeds
100g sunflower seeds
2 tbsp chia seeds
4 tbsp sesame seeds

In the food processor blend the banana, coconut oil, tahini, salt and cinnamon, until you have a paste. Add the rest of the ingredients and pulse for another minute. Grease a roasting tin or square cake tin with coconut oil. Pour the mixture out onto the greased tin and place in the freezer for 1 hour. Remove it from the freezer, cut into bars and transfer to the fridge.

These bars will last for 1 week in the fridge.

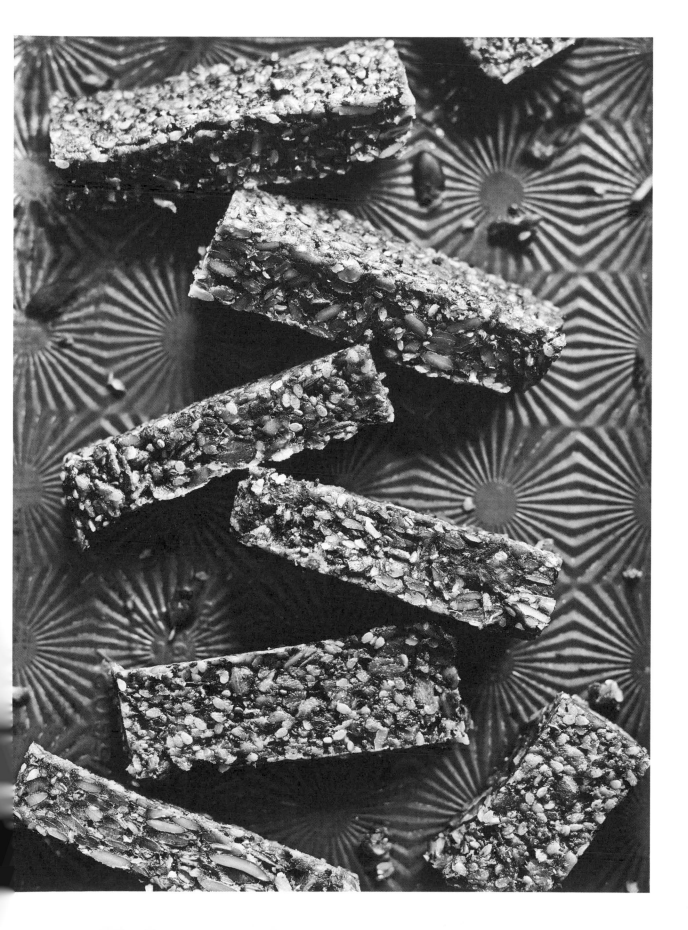

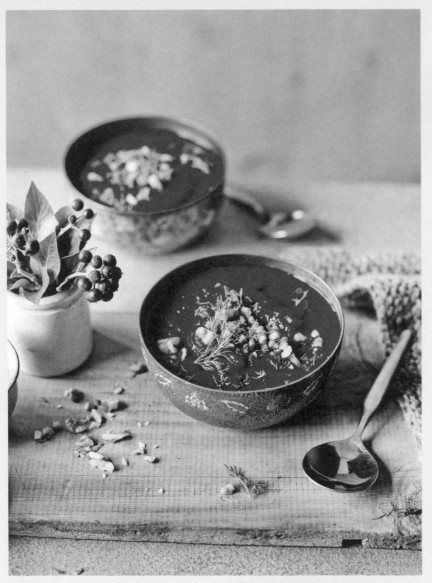

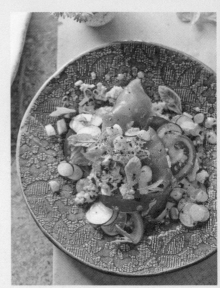

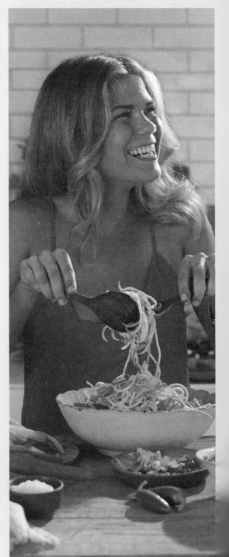

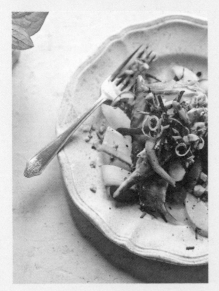

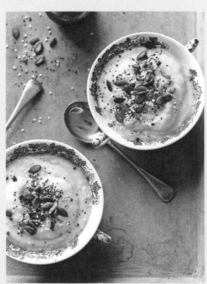

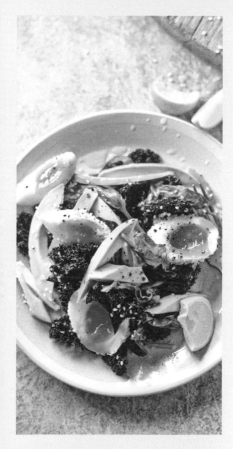

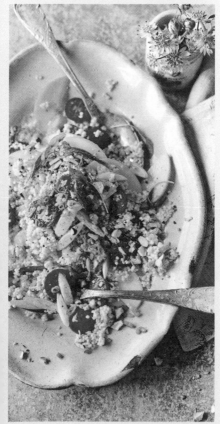

soups
and
light
salads

green gazpacho

This tastes like summer, and ticks every box: light, healthy, dairy free and, most importantly, delicious. The clean taste of cucumber and mint pairs beautifully with the creaminess of coconut, and a lovely textured crunch comes from the flaked almonds.

serves 2–3

1 cucumber, roughly chopped
1 yellow pepper, deseeded and roughly chopped
1 clove garlic, crushed
2 avocados, peeled, stoned and roughly chopped
5 spring onions, roughly chopped
1 handful fresh mint leaves
1 tbsp cider vinegar
200ml coconut milk
200ml water
2 tbsp olive oil
1 green chilli, deseeded
2 tsp sea salt
1 large grind pepper

1 tsp cayenne pepper, to serve
2 tbsp flaked almonds, to serve

Put all the ingredients except the cayenne and almonds into a blender, and blend until smooth. Sprinkle over the cayenne and almond flakes, and serve chilled.

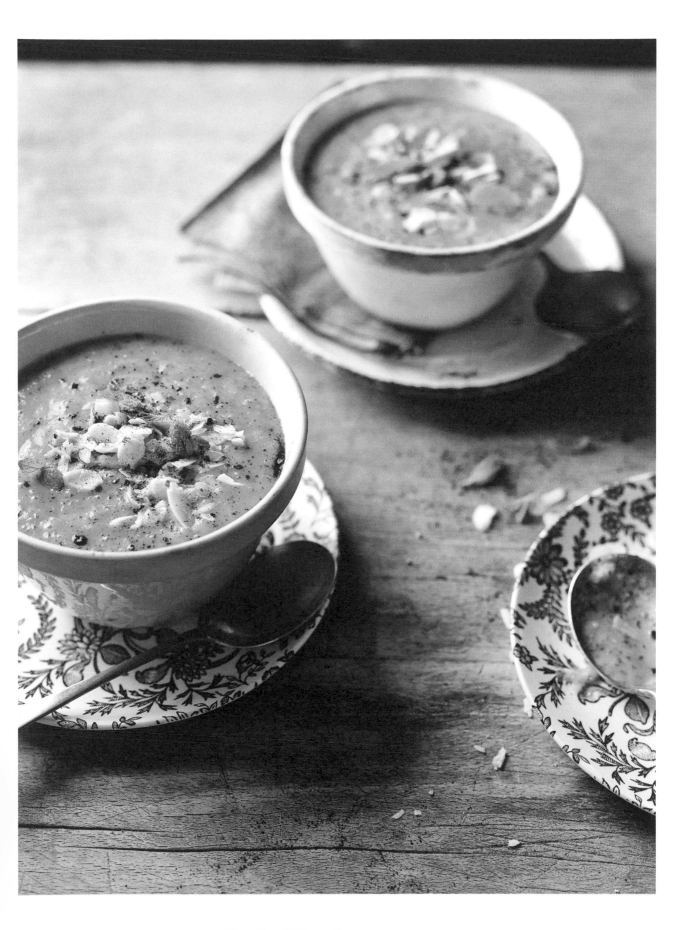

celeriac and parsnip soup with seed mix

This gorgeous root veg soup is so creamy and nourishing. The seedy mix scattered over the top gives an omega-3 crunch to this masterpiece.

serves 4–6

1 tbsp coconut oil or butter
1 white onion, finely chopped
2 pinches salt
3 large or 5 small parsnips, peeled and cut into chunks
1 celeriac, peeled and cut into chunks
500ml bone broth, or chicken or vegetable stock
1 x 400ml can coconut milk
5 tbsp pumpkin seeds
2 tbsp sesame seeds
1 tbsp chia seeds
2 tsp chilli flakes

Heat the coconut oil or butter in a large saucepan over a low heat for 1 minute, then add the onion and a pinch of salt. Sauté for 5 minutes.

Add the parsnip and celeriac to the onions and sauté for 3 minutes, then pour in the broth or stock, coconut milk and add another big pinch of salt. Bring to a simmer and cook for 30 minutes, then blend with a hand blender.

Mix the seeds and chilli flakes in a bowl, and scatter them over the top of the soup when you are ready to serve it.

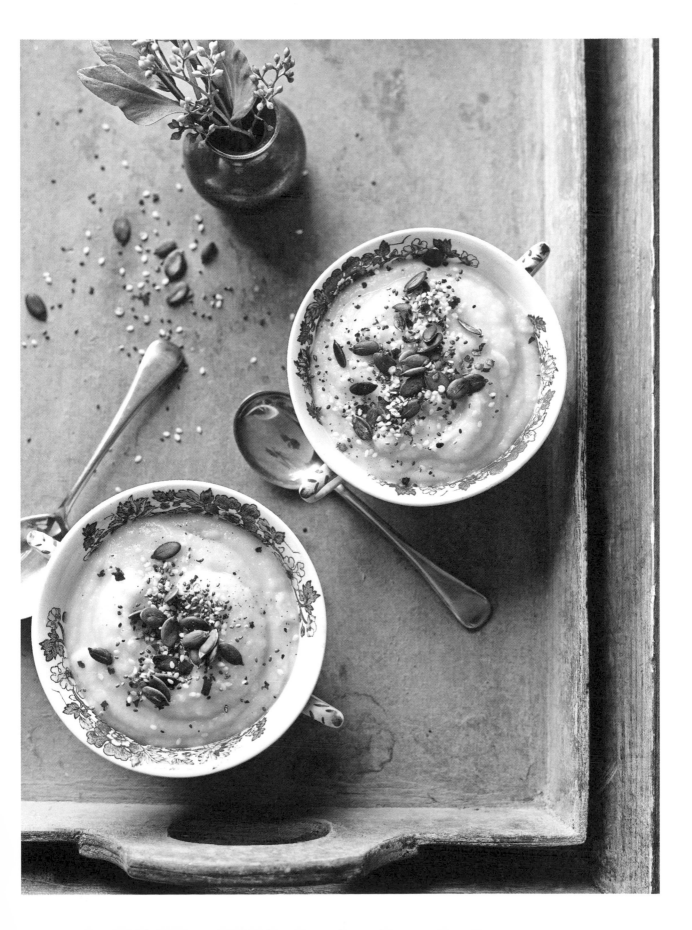

beetroot and sweet potato soup

This is such a comforting, earthy soup. I love to make a batch of this at the beginning of the week and enjoy it all week long. Topped with omega-3-rich walnuts and fresh dill, it's bound to lighten anyone's mood.

serves 4

3 sweet potatoes, peeled and cut into bite-size chunks
3 beetroots, peeled and cut into bite-size chunks
2 tbsp coconut oil, melted
1 tbsp ground cumin
1 onion, finely chopped
500ml bone broth, chicken or vegetable stock
200ml water
5 tbsp walnuts, chopped
10g finely chopped fresh dill
salt and pepper

Rub the chunks of sweet potato and beetroot in 1 tablespoon coconut oil, the cumin and a grind of salt and pepper.

Heat 1 tablespoon coconut oil in a large saucepan over a medium heat for 1 minute, add the onion and sauté with a pinch of salt for 5 minutes. Throw in the sweet potato and beetroot and sauté for 3 minutes, stirring constantly so nothing burns, then add the broth or stock, and the water. Simmer for 30 minutes, then purée with a hand blender, and serve scattered with walnuts and dill.

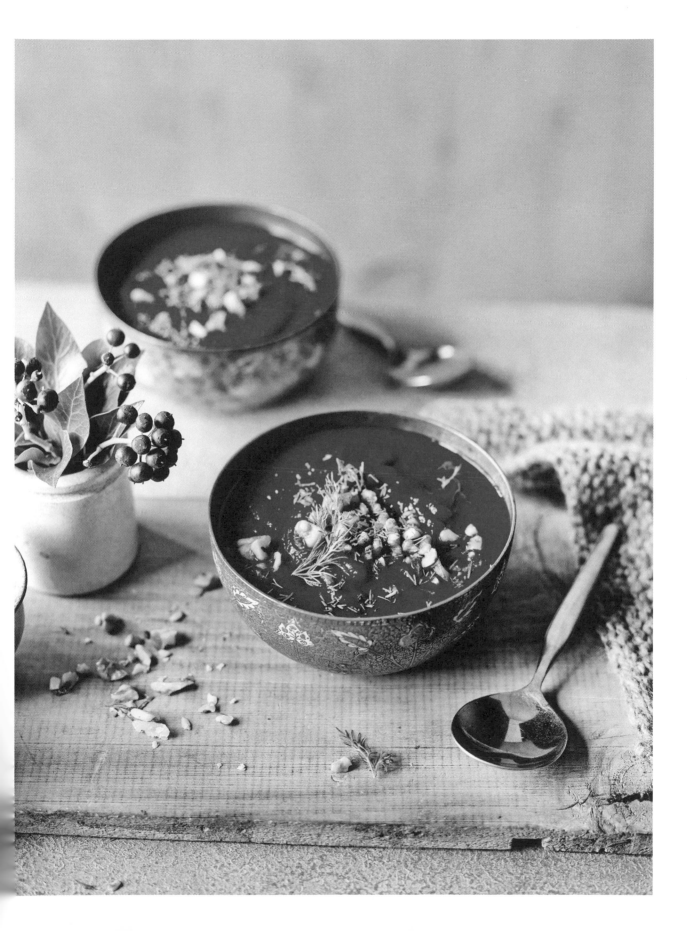

butternut and coconut soup

The only thing I like about summer being over is soup season. Try to make your own stock or buy it fresh – you will taste the difference. This soup is about to become a staple for you.

serves 6

1 butternut squash
2 tbsp coconut oil or butter, melted
pinch sea salt
1 tbsp fresh rosemary
1 white onion, finely chopped
1 x 400ml can coconut milk
250ml boiling water, chicken stock or bone broth

2 tsp chilli flakes, to serve

Preheat the oven to 200°C/400°F/Gas mark 6.

Cut the squash in half, rub the cut sides in 1 tablespoon melted coconut oil or butter and sea salt, wrap each half in foil and bake in the oven for 30–40 minutes, or until cooked through.

Scoop out the squash flesh with a spoon and set aside. In a saucepan, heat 1 tablespoon coconut oil or butter with the rosemary for 1 minute over a low heat, then add the chopped onion. Sauté for 5 minutes, then add the coconut milk, squash and boiling water, stock or broth. Cook for 10 minutes over a low heat and serve with a sprinkle of chilli flakes.

lentil and tomato soup

This soup is so nourishing. It's super simple, too, making great use of store-cupboard basics. I like to use split lentils, as they don't require soaking and give a gorgeous rich texture. The garlic gives it some spice as well as a nice boost to the immune system.

serves 2

1 tsp ground cumin
1 tsp ground coriander
1 tbsp coconut oil or butter
1 red onion, finely diced
2 cloves garlic, crushed
100g red lentils
300ml chicken or vegetable stock
1 x 400g can chopped tomatoes
natural yoghurt and fresh coriander, to serve
salt and pepper

In a large pan, dry-fry the cumin and coriander over a medium heat for 30 seconds, then add the coconut oil or butter. Pop the diced onion in with a pinch of salt, and sauté for 5 minutes.

Throw in the garlic and cook, stirring, for 1 minute then add the lentils. Add the stock and tomatoes. Bring to a simmer and let the soup cook for 20 minutes. Season with salt and pepper at the end of the cooking time.

Serve topped with a dollop of yoghurt and some fresh coriander.

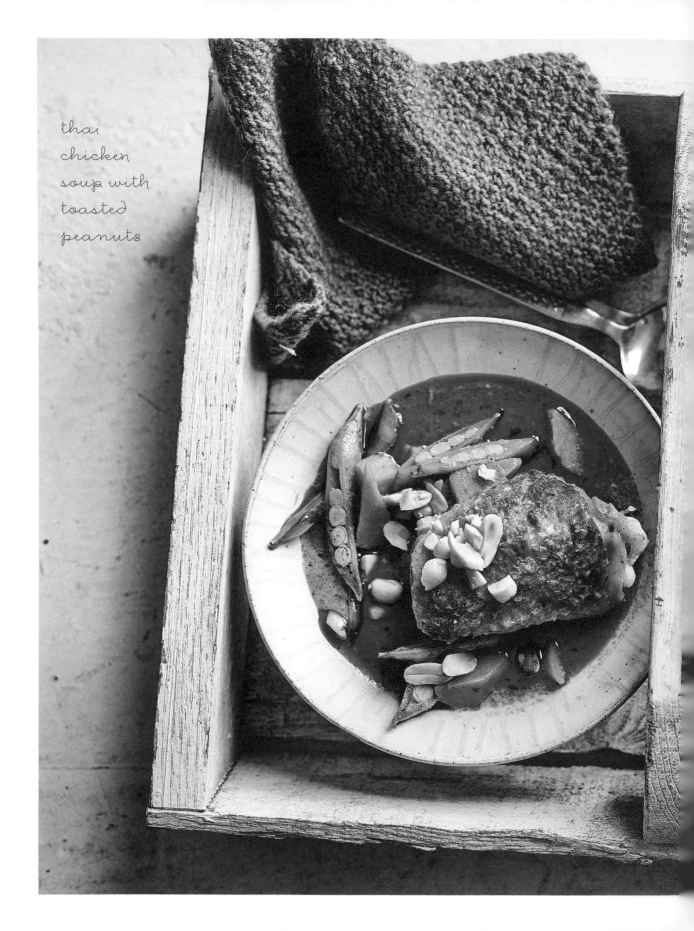

thai
chicken
soup with
toasted
peanuts

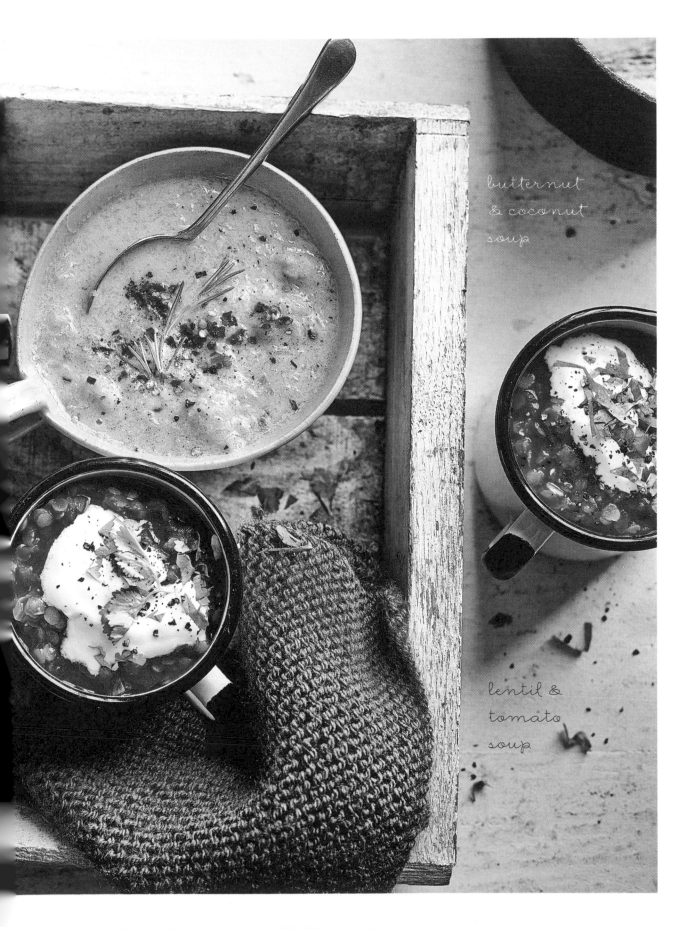

butternut
& coconut
soup

lentil &
tomato
soup

thai chicken soup with toasted peanuts

serves 2

1 tbsp coconut oil
4 chicken thighs,
  skin on and
  bone in
1 tsp freshly grated
  ginger
1 clove garlic,
  crushed
1 sweet potato,
  peeled and cut
  into 1cm cubes
2 tbsp red curry
  paste
1 tsp smoked
  paprika
1 x 400ml can
  coconut milk
300ml chicken
  stock or water
1 tbsp gluten-free
  tamari, soy sauce
  or Liquid Aminos
juice of 1 lime
1 handful peanuts
200g sugarsnap
  peas, halved
salt and pepper

This soup has a great kick from the curry paste, which teams well with the creamy coconut milk. Sugarsnap peas have to be one of my favourite veggies, and they give this soup some sweetness and a nice crunch.

Heat the coconut oil in a large saucepan over a medium heat. Sprinkle a pinch of salt over the chicken, and rub in the ginger and garlic. Throw the chicken into the pan and cook for 10 minutes, turning so it browns on all sides, then remove it from the pan and put it to one side.

Put the sweet potato into the same pan, and cook for 10 minutes, adding more coconut oil if you need to. Add the curry paste and smoked paprika, and cook while stirring for a further minute.

Pour over the coconut milk and stock or water, and bring to a simmer. Pop the chicken back into the pan and add the soy sauce, tamari or Liquid Aminos. Simmer for 10–15 minutes, until the chicken is cooked, then squeeze in the lime juice.

In a dry frying pan, toast the peanuts until lightly browned. Serve the soup with the toasted peanuts sprinkled over, and sugarsnap peas thrown in.

four amazing jam jar salad dressings

A dressing is what gives life to a salad. And when you do it healthily, you have all the nutritious benefits, too. Cider vinegar is amazing for digestion, and really gives your skin the glow. For all the dressings, simply put the ingredients in a jam jar, shake it with the lid on, and pour over your salad.

each dressing serves 8

classic lemon dressing
8 tbsp olive oil
juice of 1 lemon
pinch salt

cider vinegar dressing
8 tbsp olive oil
3 tbsp cider vinegar
pinch salt
pinch ground pepper

French dressing
8 tbsp olive oil
½ garlic clove, crushed
pinch salt
1 tsp Dijon mustard
2 tbsp cider vinegar

honey and mustard dressing
8 tbsp olive oil
pinch salt
1 tsp English mustard
1 tbsp runny honey

green goddess bowl

serves 2

50g kale, thinly
  shredded
1 tbsp coconut oil
100g spinach
4 eggs
3 tbsp sesame
  seeds
1 avocado
3 tbsp olive oil
1 tbsp cider vinegar
1 tsp Dijon mustard
1 lime, cut into
  wedges, to serve
salt and pepper

This is a bowl of total green goodness. Inspired by lazy breakfasts in Bondi Beach, this dish will instantly transform you into a goddess. Thanks to the vitamin-packed kale and the skin-saving avocado, you will be bouncing out the door after this number.

Heat the coconut oil in a pan over medium heat. Add the shredded kale with a pinch of salt and sauté for 4 minutes.

Put the spinach in a bowl and pour just-boiled water from a kettle over it to cover, then strain through a sieve. Mix this through the kale, and set aside.

Half-fill a pan with boiling water, and gently drop in the eggs one by one (make sure the water covers them). Boil the eggs for 5 minutes (for runny) and up to 9 minutes (for hard-boiled). Remove the eggs from the pan, and run them under cold water to cool. Crack the shell all around gently with a spoon, and keep the egg under a little cold running water while you peel off the shell.

Spread the sesame seeds out on a plate, mixed with a pinch of salt. Rub the eggs evenly in the sesame seed mixture.

Cut open the avocado, scoop out the flesh and cut it into chunks. Shake the olive oil, vinegar and mustard in a jam jar.

Divide all the components between two bowls, squeeze over the lime wedges and drizzle over the dressing from the jam jar.

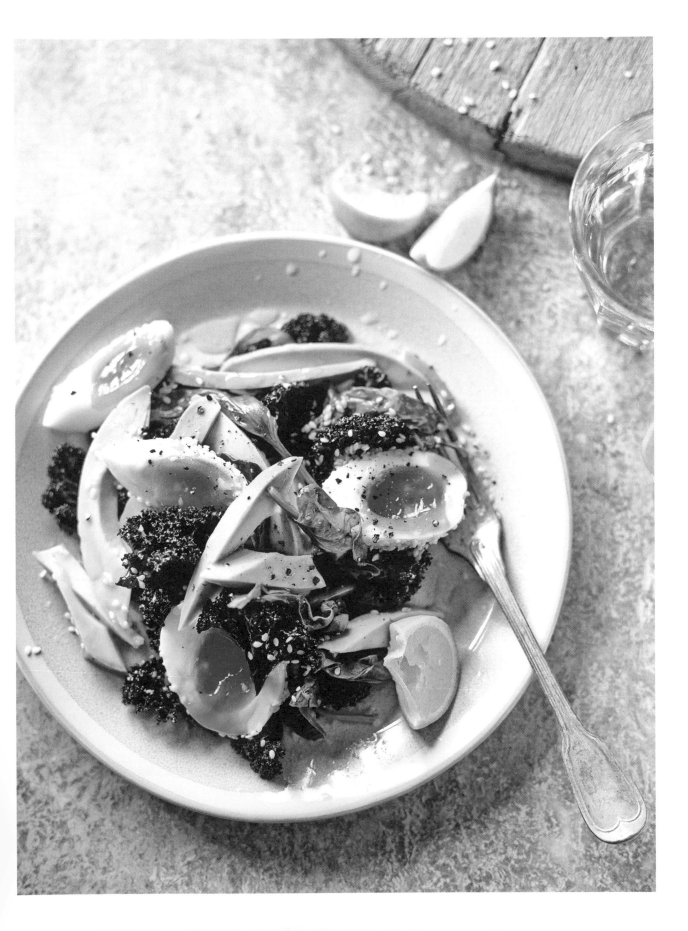

halloumi salad with kale and strawberry vinaigrette

I massage the kale before using it, as it can be quite a robust leaf, and this makes it easier to digest the iron and vitamins it contains. The saltiness of the halloumi perfectly complements the sweet acidity of strawberry, and bulks up the salad amazingly.

serves 2

2 tbsp coconut oil
½ red onion, thinly sliced
1 bunch kale, leaves massaged and sliced lengthways into strips
pinch salt
6 strawberries, hulled and cut into tiny chunks
2 tbsp water
juice of 1 lemon
1 tbsp cider vinegar
1 tbsp olive oil
200g halloumi, cut into 1cm slices
2 tbsp sesame seeds, to serve

Heat 1 tablespoon coconut oil in a large wok over a high heat for 1 minute. Add the onion and sauté for 3 minutes, then add the kale and a pinch of salt, and stir-fry for another 3 minutes. Set aside.

Put the strawberries in a pan with the water, lemon juice, vinegar and olive oil and heat over a low heat. Mash down the berries to form a purée, and put this in a small jam jar to cool.

Heat the remaining tablespoon of coconut oil in a frying pan over a high heat, then fry the halloumi for 1 minute on each side.

Grab two serving plates and pop the kale and halloumi on top, then pour over the dressing and scatter with sesame seeds.

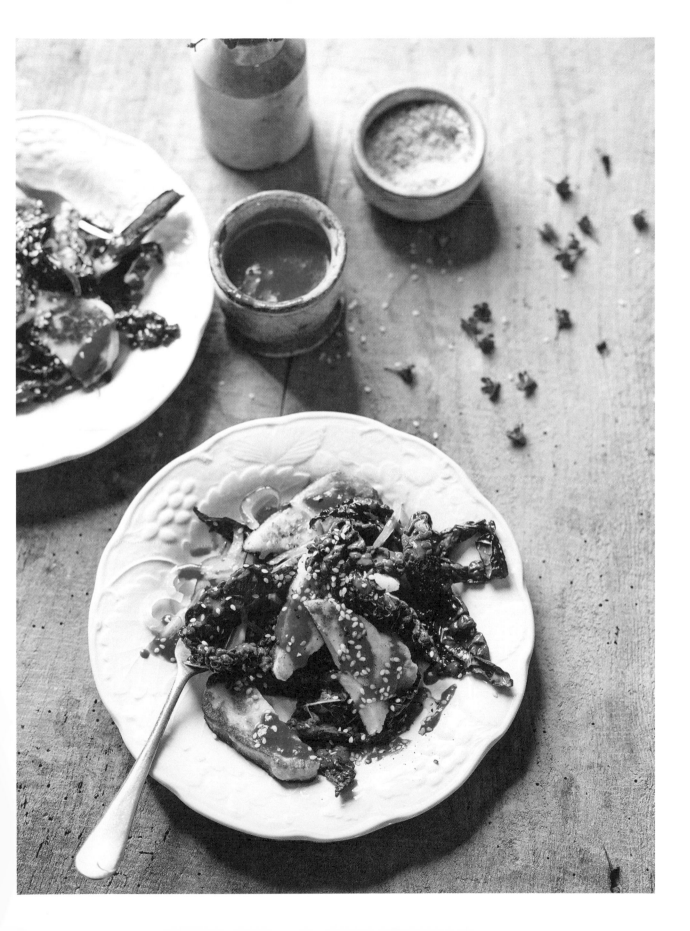

superfood crispy broccoli

serves 4 as a side

200ml water
300g tenderstem
  broccoli
1 tbsp coconut oil
3 tbsp olive oil
zest and juice of
  1 lemon
1 tsp chilli flakes
3 tbsp pumpkin
  seeds
3 tbsp goji berries
salt and pepper

This side salad is not your typical steamed broccoli. No, it has a lot of crunch and a whole host of superfoods piled in. We all know broccoli is good for us, but this salad takes it to another level with antioxidant-packed goji berries, vitamin C–rich chilli and essential fatty acids from the trusty coconut.

Boil the water in the kettle. Put the broccoli florets into a large saucepan, and pour over the boiling water and add a pinch of salt. Put a lid on the pan, and keep it at a simmer over a low heat. Allow to steam for 4 minutes, then drain and immediately run the broccoli under ice-cold water.

Heat a griddle pan over a high heat with ½ tablespoon coconut oil. Grill the broccoli for 4 minutes, turning every minute or so to ensure that it cooks evenly.

Put the broccoli in a bowl with the olive oil, a pinch of salt and a good grind of pepper. Add the lemon zest and juice, and give everything a good stir.

Heat the remaining coconut oil in a frying pan and toast the chilli flakes with the pumpkin seeds for 2 minutes, then toss this over the broccoli with the goji berries.

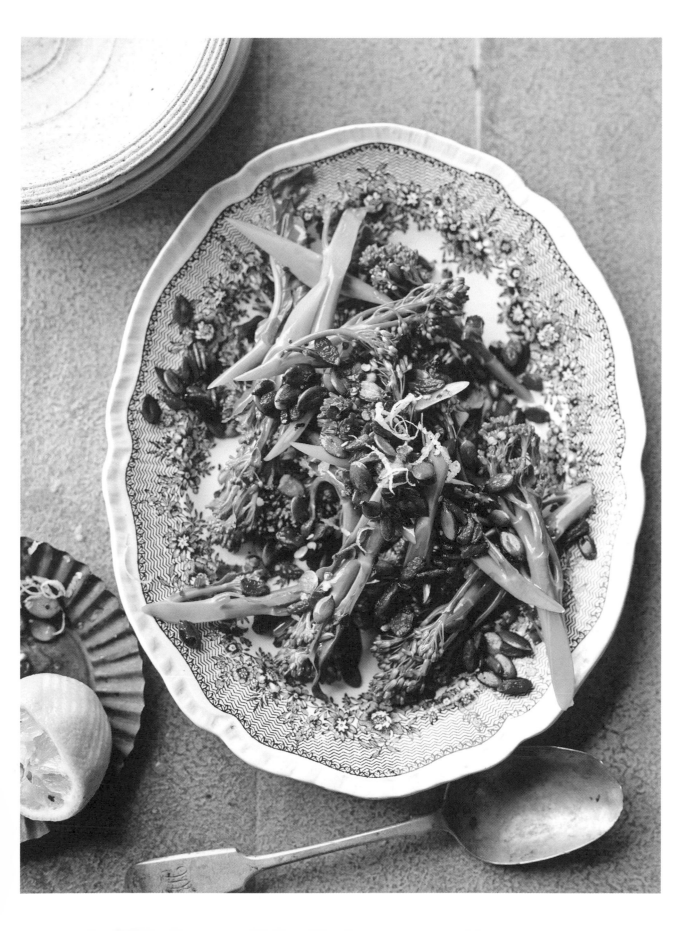

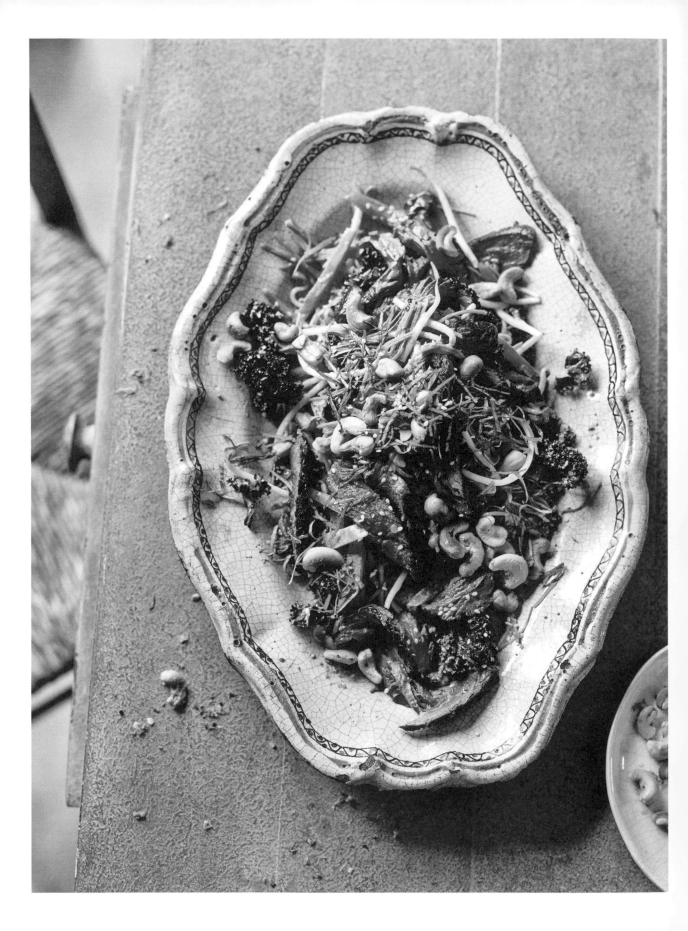

thai beef salad with salt and pepper cashews

This salad was created for my mum, and without a doubt this is the only dish she will order when we go for Thai. Creamy tahini teamed with the salt and pepper cashews gives this salad an exhilarating flavour. I like to keep my beef raw in the middle, for a bit of a modern twist on a conventional Thai salad.

Grind some salt and pepper over the steaks and leave on one side.

In a medium frying pan heat 1 teaspoon coconut oil with ½ teaspoon salt and ½ teaspoon freshly ground pepper. Throw in the cashew nuts, toss well and cook over a medium heat for 5 minutes. Stir the lime zest into the nuts and set aside.

In a glass, whisk the juice of the lime with the garlic, ginger, tahini, chilli, and tamari, soy sauce or Liquid Aminos.

Put the kale and red pepper in a bowl. Pour the dressing over the kale salad, massaging the dressing into the kale so it wilts. Throw in the grated carrot and beansprouts.

Heat a griddle pan over a high heat. When it's hot, sear the steaks for 3 minutes on each side. Let the beef rest for a few minutes, then slice it finely and layer it over the salad. Sprinkle over the sesame seeds and cashew nuts. Finely chop the basil and coriander and throw them over the top.

serves 2

2 rib-eye steaks (or other favourite cut)
1 tsp coconut oil
50g cashew nuts
zest and juice of 1 lime
1 large clove garlic, crushed
1 tbsp freshly grated ginger
2 tbsp tahini
1 red chilli, chopped, and deseeded if you like it less spicy
2 tsp gluten-free tamari, soy sauce or Liquid Aminos
50g kale, cut into ½cm strips
1 red pepper, cut into ½cm strips
2 carrots, grated
50g beansprouts
1 tbsp sesame seeds
10g fresh basil
10g fresh coriander
salt and pepper

spring salad: grapefruit, smashed egg and asparagus

serves 2

1 small cos lettuce,
 stalk removed and
 leaves separated
1 ruby grapefruit,
 skin and pith
 removed, sliced
 lengthways into
 1cm slices
1 bunch asparagus,
 ends removed
zest and juice of
 1 lemon
1 handful fresh
 coriander, finely
 chopped
4 eggs
2 tsp smoked
 paprika
2 tsp chilli flakes
3 tsp olive oil
salt

I love spring. It's my birthday season and, more importantly, it's spring fruit and vegetable season! Asparagus is great for detoxing the body, grapefruit is bursting with vitamin C and the eggs provide you with a protein kick.

Arrange the lettuce leaves on two serving plates. Lay the grapefruit slices over the lettuce.

Steam the asparagus spears for 5 minutes, then throw them over the salad. Sprinkle the lemon zest and juice and the coriander over the salad too.

Half-fill a pan with boiling water, and gently drop in the eggs one by one (make sure the water covers them). Boil the eggs for 5 minutes (for runny) and up to 9 minutes (for hard-boiled). Remove the eggs from the pan, and run them under cold water to cool. Crack the shell all around gently with a spoon, and keep the eggs under a little cold running water while you peel off the shell.

Spread the paprika, a pinch of salt and the chilli flakes over a plate, and rub the eggs into this mixture until they are evenly covered.

Cut the eggs in half over the salad, drizzle over the olive oil, add a pinch of salt, and eat immediately.

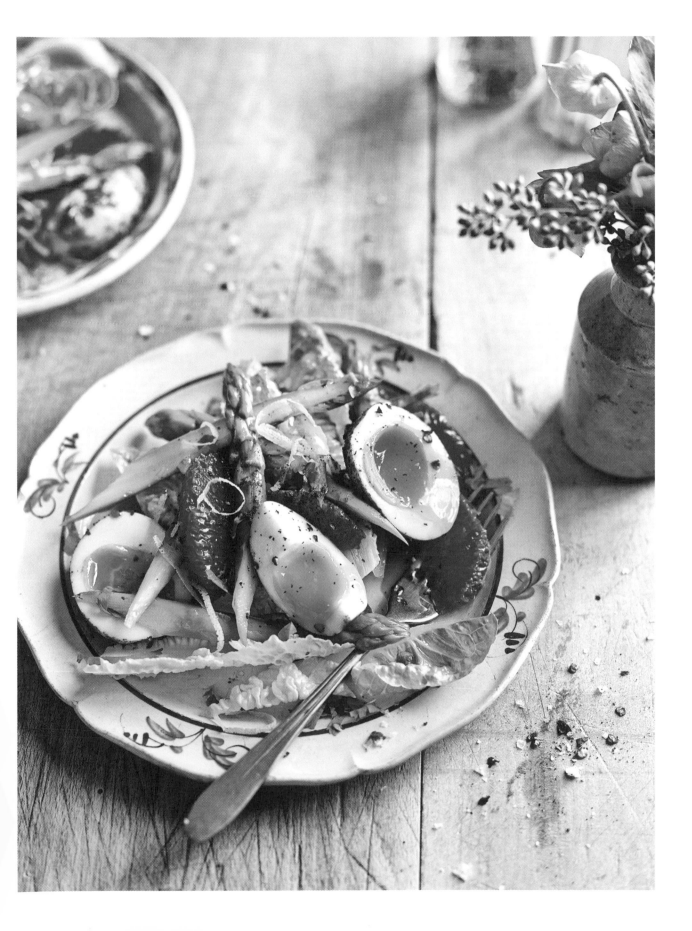

summer salad: grilled nectarine, parma ham and runner bean

This is my summer salad, and it beautifully marries the sweet flavour of nectarine with the salty prosciutto. The texture of the cured meat alongside its softer counterparts really allows this summer salad to live up to its name.

serves 2

150g runner beans, sliced
2 nectarines
30g watercress
30g rocket
100g Parma ham
50g feta cheese, sliced
2 tbsp sesame seeds (optional)
3 tbsp Honey and Mustard Dressing (see page 127)
salt and pepper

Pop the beans into a pan with a little water and a pinch of salt, and steam for 5 minutes.

Cut the nectarines into eighths, put them on a griddle pan over a medium heat, and griddle for 2 minutes on each side.

Put the watercress and rocket into a bowl and mix them together. Scatter the rest of the ingredients over the top, then pour over the dressing and finish with some cracked black pepper.

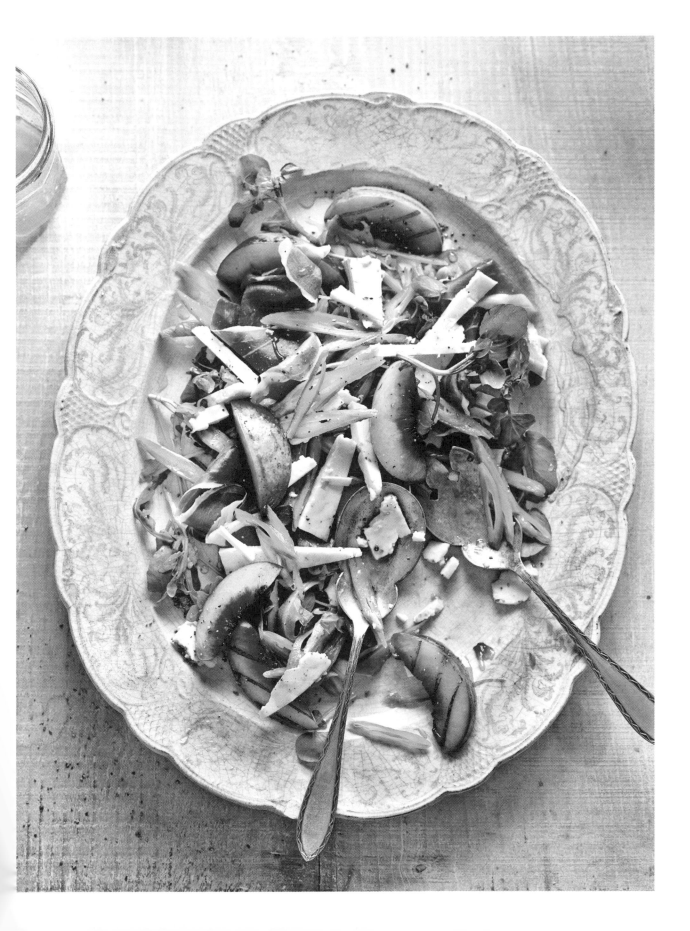

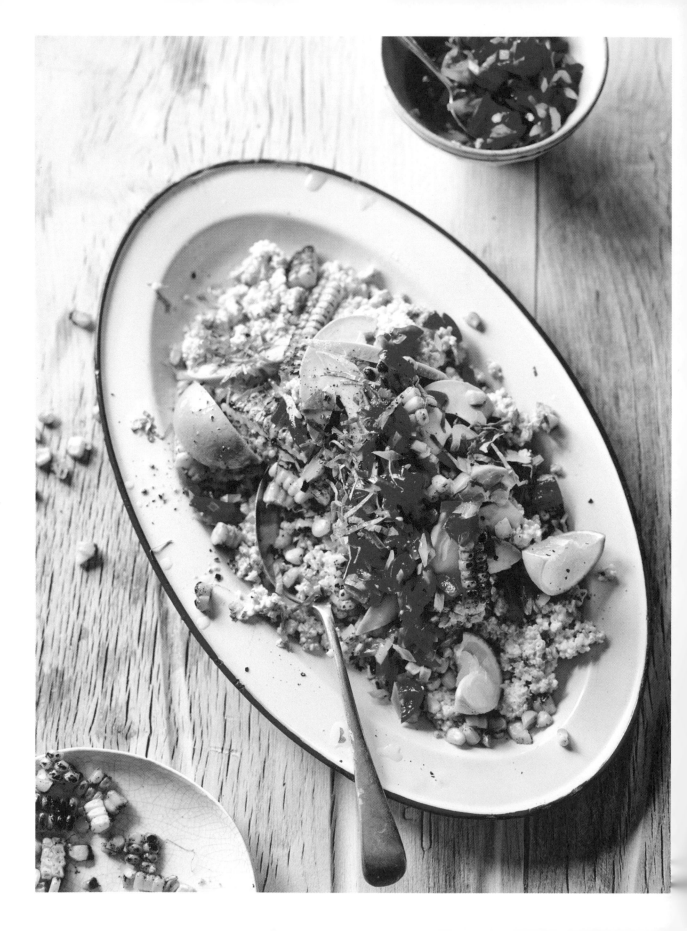

autumn salad: mexican bbq grilled corn and quinoa, with chilli salsa

As autumn kicks in and the temperature drops, I prefer a salad with a bit of a kick. Paprika and cayenne take to quinoa amazingly, giving the zingy heat I crave. And because the corn is barbecued in coconut oil, it gives you some extra-nutritious goodness.

Put the quinoa in a saucepan with the water and a pinch of salt. Bring it to the boil, then turn the heat down and let it gently simmer for 12–15 minutes, or until all the water has been absorbed.

Heat a griddle pan over a medium heat. Meanwhile, mix the melted coconut oil or butter, smoked paprika, cayenne and a pinch of salt and freshly ground pepper. Brush the spiced oil evenly over both corn cobs. Wrap them in foil and griddle them, rotating every few minutes, for 20 minutes, or until cooked. Unwrap the corn, let it cool, then use a knife to cut the corn away from the cob.

To make the salsa, put the tomatoes and pepper into a bowl, then dress them with the cider vinegar, olive oil and a pinch of salt.

Mix the chopped coriander through the quinoa with the yoghurt, lime juice, a pinch of salt and some freshly ground pepper. Throw the corn over the quinoa, then the salsa, and finally scatter the avocado chunks on top.

serves 2

125g quinoa
200ml water
2 tbsp coconut oil
  or butter, melted
1 tsp smoked
  paprika
1 tsp cayenne
  pepper
2 corn cobs, outer
  leaves removed
200g cherry
  tomatoes, diced
  into tiny squares
1 red pepper, diced
  into tiny squares
1 green pepper,
  diced into tiny
  squares
2 tbsp cider
  vinegar
1 tbsp olive oil
100g fresh
  coriander, finely
  chopped
6 tbsp Greek
  yoghurt
juice of 1 lime
1 avocado, peeled,
  stoned and cut
  into chunks
salt and pepper

winter salad: shaved brussels sprouts, cauliflower rice and pomegranate

This salad is the perfect way to jazz up your sprouts. I love the richness of pomegranates teamed with the crunchy pecan nuts. Shaving your sprouts makes them soak up all the juices and gives them a fun texture.

serves 2

100g Brussels sprouts
½ cauliflower, stalk removed and roughly chopped
2 tbsp coconut oil
zest and juice of 1 lemon
½ pomegranate
3 tbsp olive oil
1 tsp mustard
1 tbsp cider vinegar
3 tbsp halved pecan nuts
salt and pepper

Shred the Brussels sprouts in a food processor or use a mandoline. Put the roughly chopped cauliflower into a food processor and process for a few minutes until you get a rice-like consistency. Heat the coconut oil and a pinch of salt in a large frying pan for 1 minute over a medium heat, then throw in the cauliflower and the sprouts. Sauté the vegetables for 3 minutes, then transfer to a bowl. Stir in the lemon zest and juice, and set aside to let this soak in.

Bash out the pomegranate seeds with a spoon, then remove the white pith and sprinkle them over the top of the veg.

In a jam jar shake the olive oil, mustard, vinegar and a pinch of salt.

Throw this over everything at the end, along with the pecans.

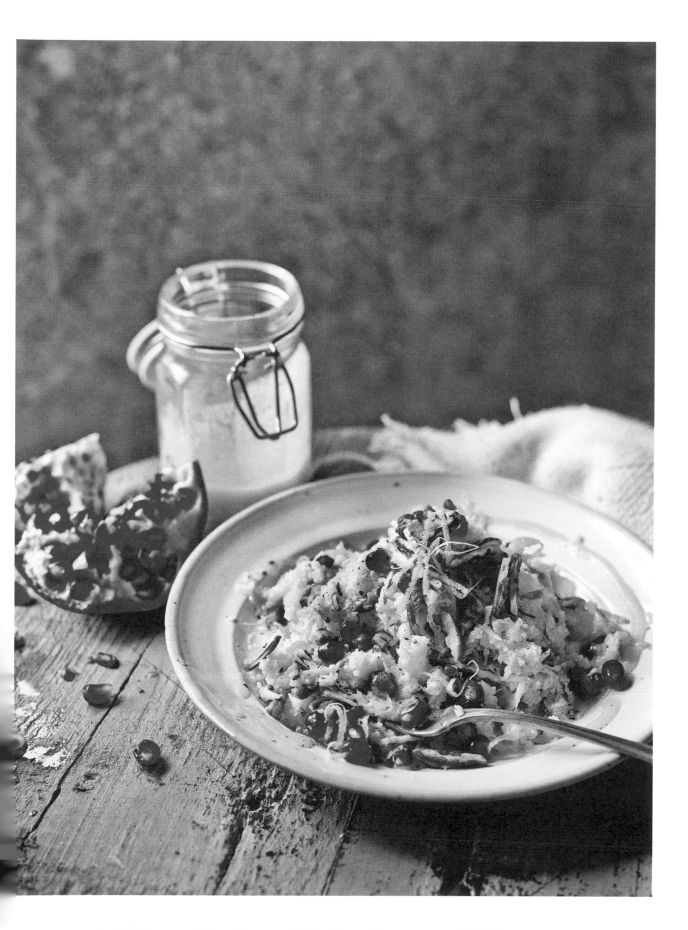

grilled chicken, roasted lemon and olive salad

This has a lovely taste of the Middle East, with protein from chicken, tang from cumin-spiced yoghurt and acidity coming from the ripe olives and burnt lemon. This recipe always reminds me of Israel.

serves 2

2 large chicken breasts
1 large clove garlic, crushed
1 tsp ground cumin
1 tbsp coconut oil or butter, melted
1 lemon
4 tbsp natural yoghurt
2 tbsp olive oil
1 cos lettuce, stalk removed and sliced lengthways into 1cm strips
10 large green olives, halved
4 tbsp pine nuts, toasted

Rub the chicken in the garlic, cumin and coconut oil or butter. Heat a griddle pan over a medium heat for a few minutes, then put the chicken on it and griddle for 6 minutes on each side, turning every minute, until the chicken is cooked through.

Zest the lemon and thoroughly mix the zest with the yoghurt and olive oil. Thinly slice the lemon and put it on the griddle alongside the chicken for a minute or so on each side.

Put the cos lettuce strips and olive halves in two serving bowls, then thinly slice the griddled chicken and scatter over the bowls of salad with the yoghurt dressing, roasted lemon and pine nuts.

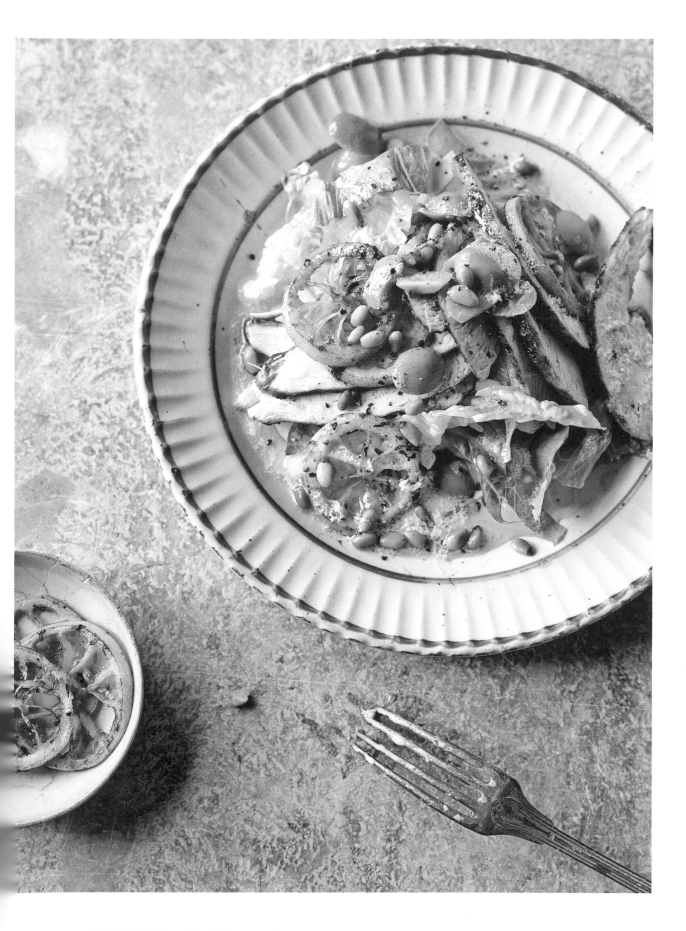

millet and sage leaf salad

Millet is so similar to quinoa, and makes a great alternative to it. It's gluten free, and it's cheaper if you're on a budget. The sage leaves will raise your levels of beta-carotene as well as vitamin A, and the spring onions and pistachios give a wonderful texture.

serves 2

125g millet
250ml boiling bone broth, chicken stock, vegetable stock or water
pinch salt
1 green apple
juice of 1 lemon
50g cherry tomatoes, halved
2 spring onions, thinly sliced
2 tbsp olive oil
1 clove garlic, crushed
1 tbsp coconut oil or butter
6 sage leaves
4 tbsp crushed pistachios

Rinse the millet in a sieve. Put the millet in a large saucepan with the boiling broth, stock or water and salt. Simmer with the lid on for 12–15 minutes, or until all the liquid is absorbed.

Thinly slice the green apple and put it in a bowl; pour the lemon juice over the apple slices to stop them from browning. Mix the tomatoes and spring onions in a bowl with the cooled millet, olive oil, garlic and apple. Heat the coconut oil or butter in a small frying pan, and fry the sage leaves for 1 minute on each side until crisp, then arrange them on top of the millet and sprinkle the pistachios over everything.

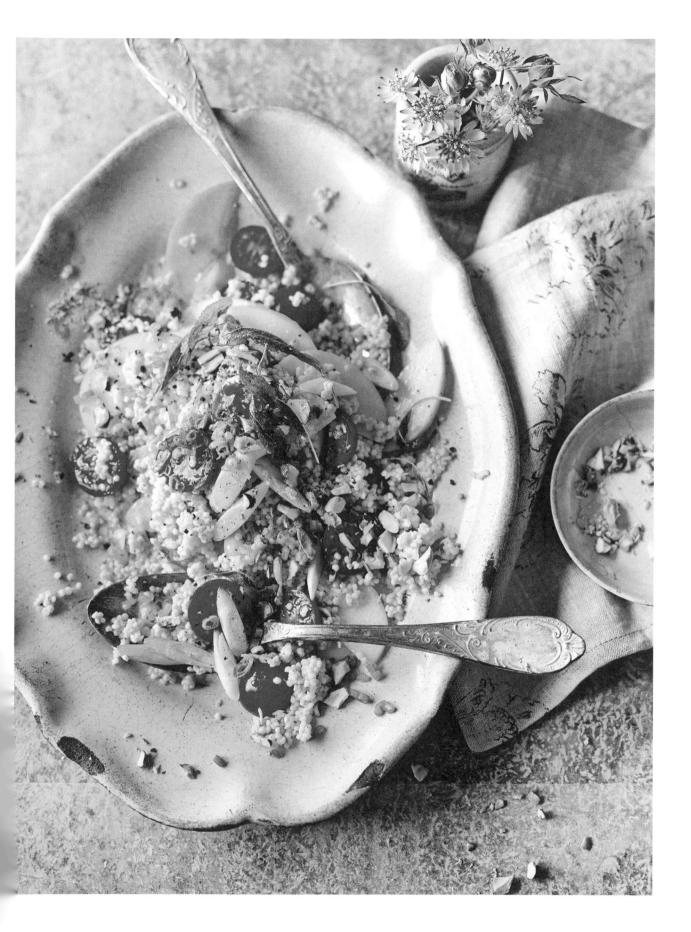

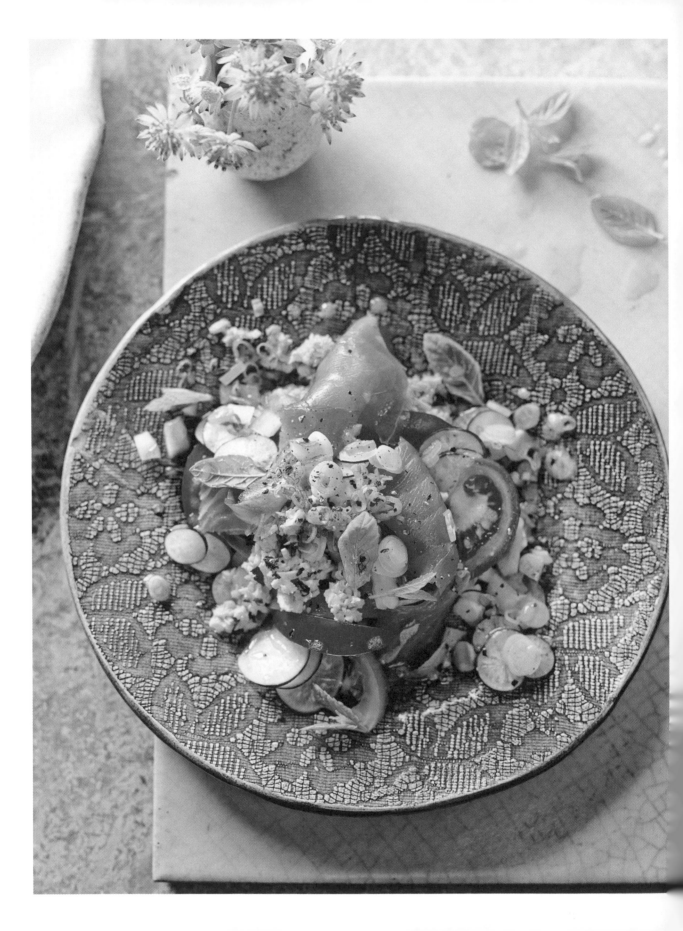

smoked salmon and fattoush salad with avocado mash

This salad has everything, and is so quick to make. Essential fats from the avocado, omega-3s from the salmon and a light crunch from the radish and cucumber make this a perfect salad for an on-the-go lifestyle.

serves 2

1 avocado, peeled and stoned
juice of 1 lime
pinch chilli flakes
30g radishes, thinly sliced
1 spring onion, thinly sliced
1 cucumber, cut into tiny cubes
2 tomatoes, quartered
1 clove garlic, crushed
zest and juice of 1 lemon
3 tbsp olive oil
2 tsp cider vinegar
300g smoked salmon

10g fresh mint leaves, to serve
salt and pepper

Put the avocado, lime juice and chilli flakes in a bowl, and mash with a fork until fairly smooth.

Put the radishes, spring onion, cucumber and tomatoes into a bowl with the garlic, a pinch each of salt and pepper, the lemon zest and juice, the olive oil and the vinegar.

Arrange the salad and the mash on a plate with the smoked salmon, and sprinkle with the mint leaves.

warm kale, chickpea and orange salad

This salad is a nutritional powerhouse, with kale – one of my favourite superfoods – working in tandem with lots of vegetable protein from the chickpeas. This evergreen dish is complemented beautifully by the zesty orange and the subtly spicy ginger.

serves 2

1 tbsp coconut oil
1 white onion, finely chopped
2 tsp ground cumin
1 tbsp freshly grated ginger
1 x 400g can chickpeas, drained
3 kale leaves, cut lengthways into thin strips
1 courgette, grated
zest and juice of 1 orange
salt and pepper

Put the coconut oil in a large frying pan with the onion and cumin, and sauté over a medium heat for 5 minutes. Add the ginger and a good grind of salt and pepper, and stir for 1 minute. Add the chickpeas and cook for a further 5 minutes, stirring constantly.

Add the kale and the courgette to the pan and cook for another 5 minutes, stirring every minute or so.

Just before serving add the orange zest and juice, and some salt and pepper. Serve warm.

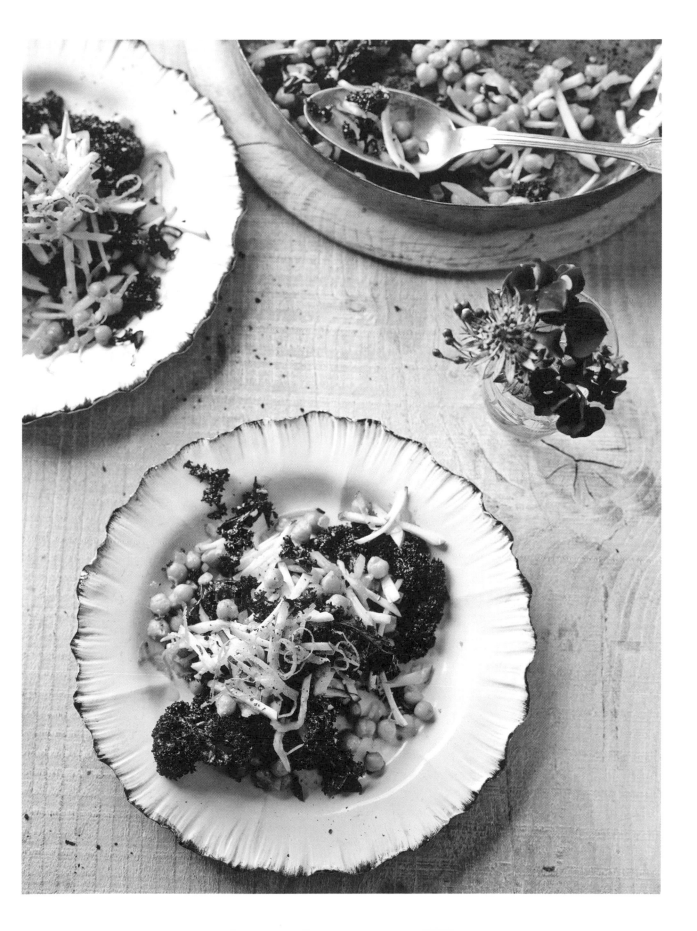

smoked mackerel salad with shaved cucumber, beetroot and orange

This simple recipe can be whipped up in minutes. It's my go-to lunch box. It's abundant in omega-3 richness thanks to the mackerel; these fatty acids will get your skin glowing all day long.

serves 2

1 orange
1 large or 2 small beetroots, grated
1 tsp olive oil
2 tbsp finely chopped chives
1 cucumber
100g cherry tomatoes, halved
30g walnuts
1 tbsp cider vinegar
2 large smoked mackerel fillets

Zest the orange. Combine the grated beetroot with the orange zest, olive oil and chopped chives. Cut the orange into eight segments, and remove the skin and pith. Peel the cucumber into ribbons with a peeler or a mandoline, and mix this with the tomatoes, walnuts, vinegar, orange and beetroot mix. Serve the salad with the mackerel on top.

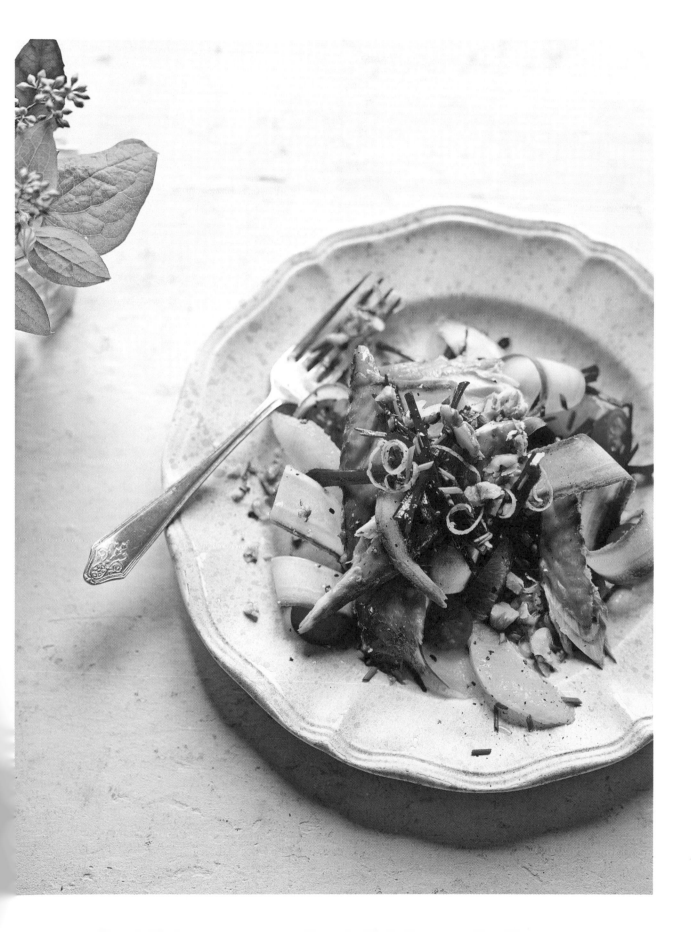

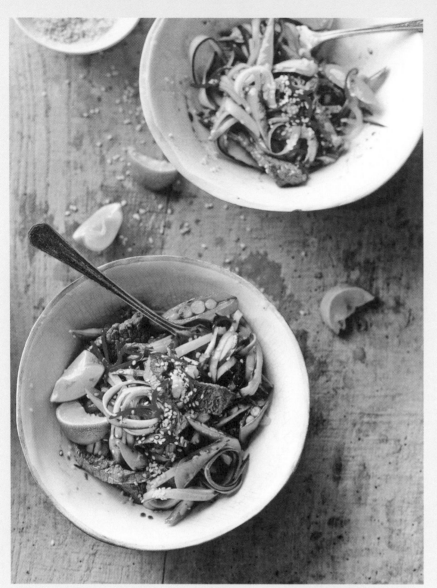
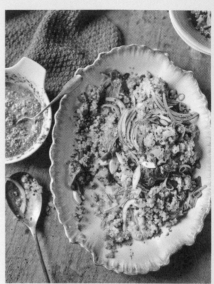
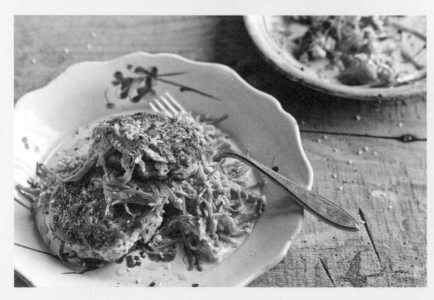
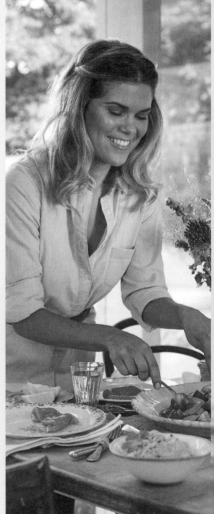

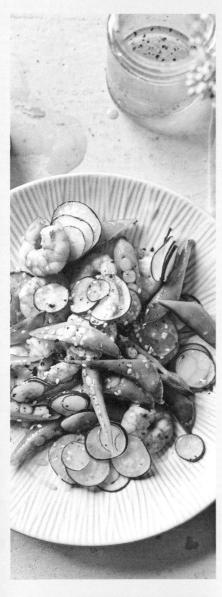

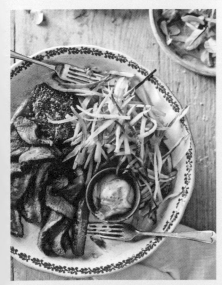

speedy suppers

spicy salmon with cucumber and yoghurt

Not only do you have the omega-3 and skin-saving benefits of spiced salmon, you also get that incredible crunch and cleanness of cucumber with the beautiful balance of yoghurt. A real winner in my eyes.

serves 2

150g natural, coconut or goat's milk yoghurt
1 lemon
3 tsp smoked paprika
1 tsp salt
2 large salmon fillets
½ a cucumber
2 tbsp chopped chives
2 tbsp sesame seeds
1 tbsp olive oil
2 tbsp coconut oil

Mix the yoghurt, lemon, paprika and salt together.
Rub 1 tablespoon of the marinade on each fish fillet.

With a peeler or mandoline, cut the cucumber into ribbons. Mix the cucumber with the chives, sesame seeds and olive oil.

In a large frying pan, heat the coconut oil for 1 minute over a high heat, then add the salmon and fry for 2–3 minutes on each side, starting with the skin side facing down.

Serve the salmon with the salad and more of the yoghurt mixture.

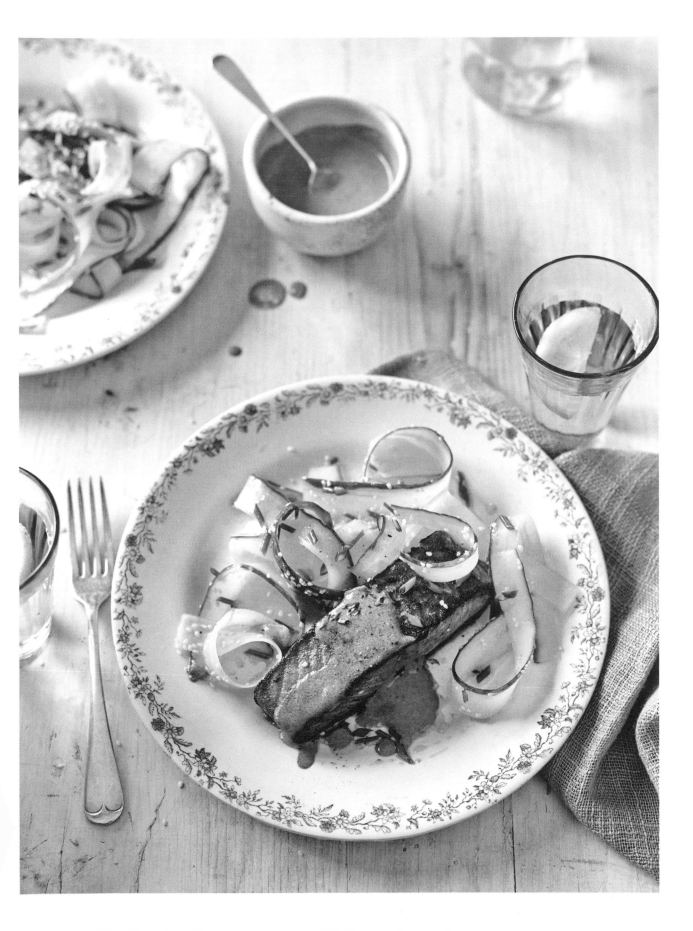

raw pad thai

serves 3

2 courgettes
1 carrot
1 yellow pepper, cut
   into thin strips
1 red pepper, cut
   into thin strips
2 spring onions,
   finely sliced
100g sugarsnap
   peas, finely
   chopped
bunch coriander,
   finely chopped
1 red chilli,
   deseeded and
   finely chopped
1 green chilli,
   deseeded and
   finely chopped
100ml coconut milk
2 tbsp tahini
juice of 2 limes
large pinch salt
1 tbsp gluten-free
   tamari, soy sauce
   or Liquid Aminos
pinch salt
2 tbsp sesame oil
3 tbsp sesame
   seeds, to serve

This is a great, raw take on Thailand's most famous export. Rawness ensures food retains its nutritional value, and the addition of red pepper sends the vitamin C levels sky-high, so this dish is great for strengthening your immune system. Loads of texture, buckets of flavour.

To make courgette noodles, spiralise or julienne the courgettes, or use a peeler to cut them into noodle or ribbon shapes. Do the same with the carrot. Put all the 'noodles' in a large serving bowl.

Add the strips of yellow and red pepper, the spring onion slices, the chopped sugarsnap peas, the coriander and the chillies.

Put the coconut milk, tahini, lime juice, tamari or soy sauce or Liquid Aminos, salt and sesame oil in a jam jar. Shake it (with the lid on!), then pour this dressing over the vegetables.

Stir the salad, then sprinkle the sesame seeds on top to serve.

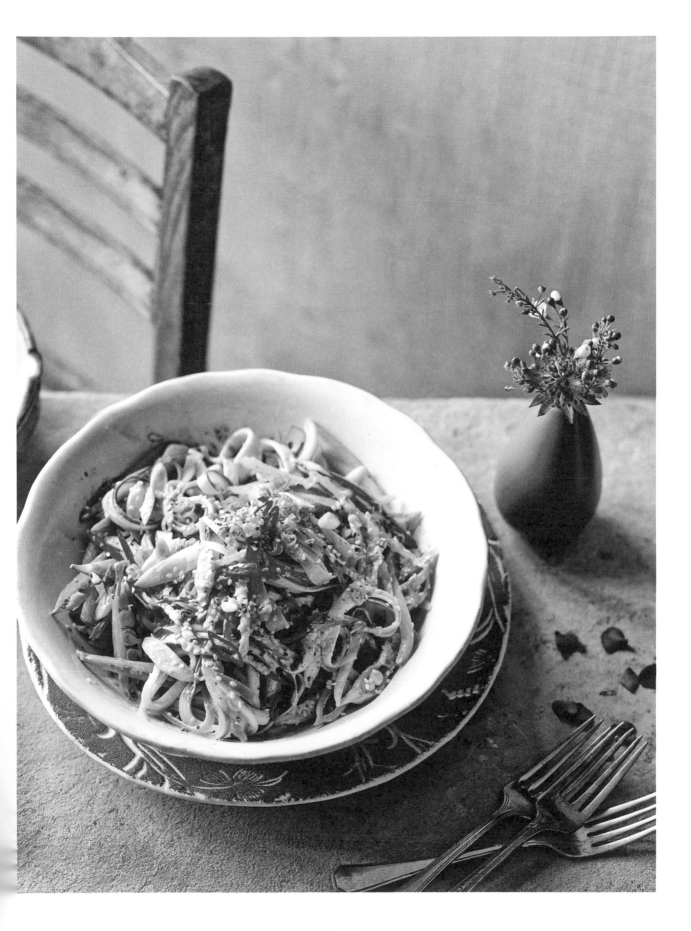

steak with parsnip chips

This is an absolute favourite of mine – it's a spin on a dish that everyone loves. My word of advice is to talk to your butcher, and always ask if the animal the meat is from has been grass fed. There are so many more nutritional benefits if this is the case. And you get to make this dish really fun with parsnip fries. Sweet, nutritious, delicious.

serves 2

2 sirloin steaks, 150–200g each
250g parsnips, peeled
4 tbsp coconut oil or butter
mustard and salad greens, to serve
salt and pepper

Preheat the oven to 220°C/425°F/Gas mark 7.

Grind pepper and salt over the steaks and leave them to marinate at room temperature.

Meanwhile, cut the parsnips into thin frites. Melt 3 tablespoons coconut oil or butter in a roasting tin, and toss the parsnips in this with a good grind of salt and pepper. Roast them in the oven until golden brown, flipping them over halfway through the cooking time. They will cook in 15–20 minutes, depending on your chip size.

Just before the chips are ready, heat a frying pan over a high heat. Add 1 tablespoon of coconut oil or butter, wait for the pan to get hot again, then cook the steaks for 2 minutes on each side. (This is for rare steak; cook another few minutes for well done.)

Serve with mustard and some salad greens.

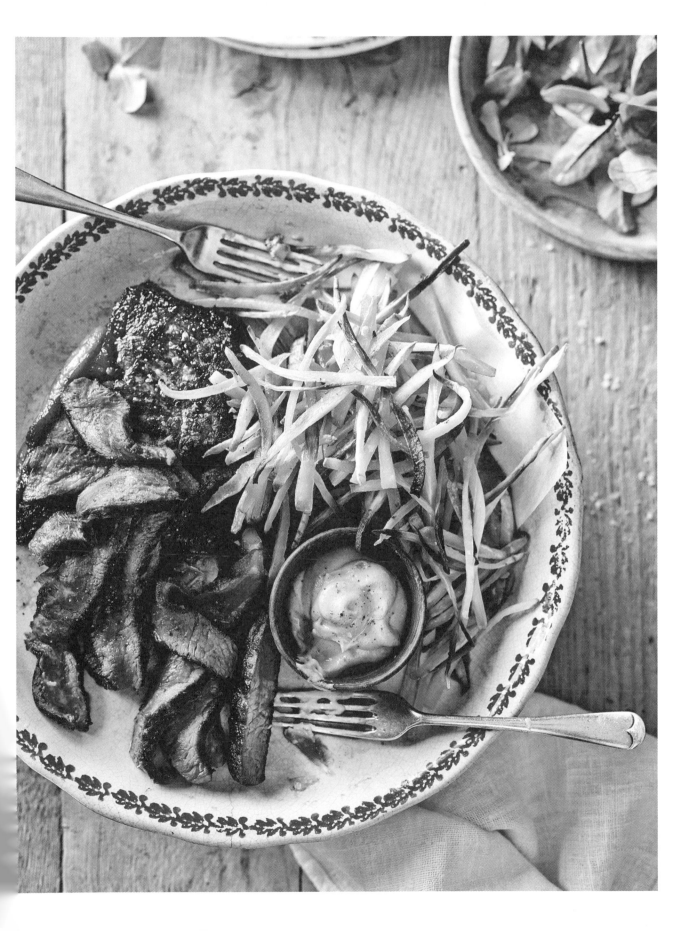

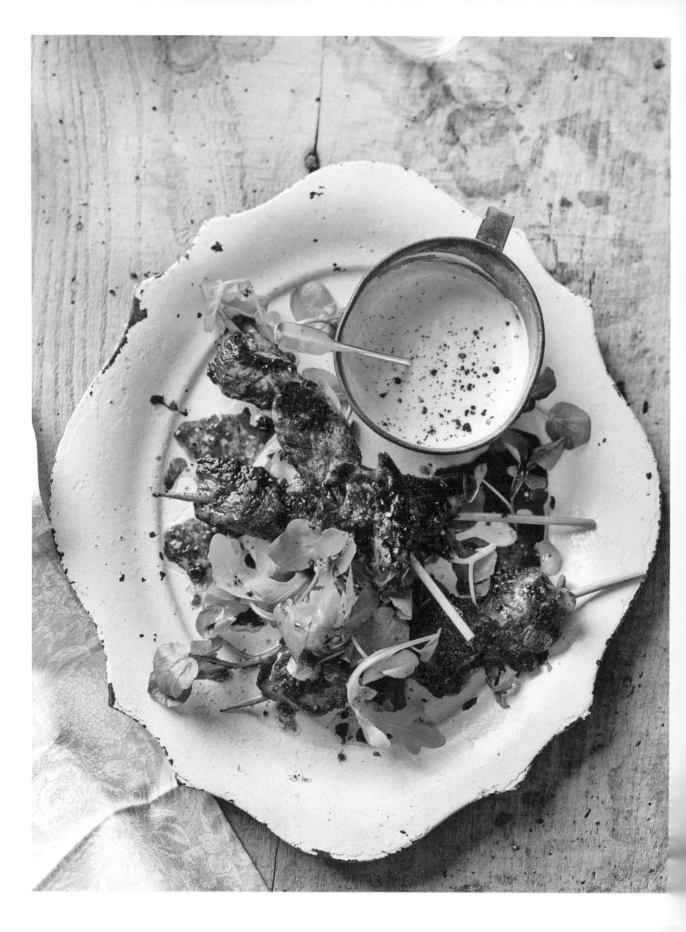

ginger beef kebabs with yoghurt and salad

On the move or in a hurry? This is the perfect answer to such situations. You have wonderful immunity boosters in the garlic and ginger, and the coconut oil doesn't denature the goodness of the other ingredients due to its high smoking point.

serves 2

1 tbsp freshly grated ginger
1 tbsp gluten-free tamari, soy sauce or Liquid Aminos
1 tbsp honey
2 cloves garlic, crushed
1 tbsp coconut oil, melted
250g beef (sirloin or rump steak), cut into 2.5cm cubes
100g natural yoghurt
3 tbsp olive oil
25g watercress
25g rocket
salt and pepper

In a bowl combine the ginger, tamari, Liquid Aminos or soy sauce, honey, 1 garlic clove and melted coconut oil, then throw the beef in. Leave this for at least 2 hours and up to 12 hours in the fridge if you can; however it will still taste great if you don't have that long.

Thread the beef on to 4 skewers. (If using wooden or bamboo skewers, soak them in water first.) Heat a griddle pan to a medium to high heat and cook the kebabs for 5 minutes, rotating every minute so they cook evenly.

Mix the yoghurt with the remaining crushed garlic, the olive oil and a grind of salt and pepper. Serve the dressing on the side, or drizzled over the watercress, rocket and kebabs.

seared prawns with a ginger sugarsnap pea salad

This is easy to make, packs a crunch and is so speedy to whip up. What more could you want? Seafood, sugarsnaps and the calcium-loaded sesame seeds make this dish a personal favourite of mine.

serves 2

300g raw king prawns
200g sugarsnap peas, ends cut off and snapped in half
100g radishes, finely sliced
1 tbsp cider vinegar
1 tbsp freshly grated ginger
1 tbsp coconut oil or butter
2 tbsp olive oil or sesame oil

2 tbsp sesame seeds
salt and pepper

Pat the prawns dry with a kitchen towel and grind salt and pepper over them.

Put the sugarsnaps in a bowl with the sliced radish. Mix the vinegar, ginger and olive or sesame oil with a pinch of salt.

Heat the coconut oil or butter in a frying pan over a high heat for 1 minute. Turn the heat down a little, and fry the prawns for 1 minute on each side until cooked through.

Plate the prawns with the salad, pour over the dressing and top with sesame seeds.

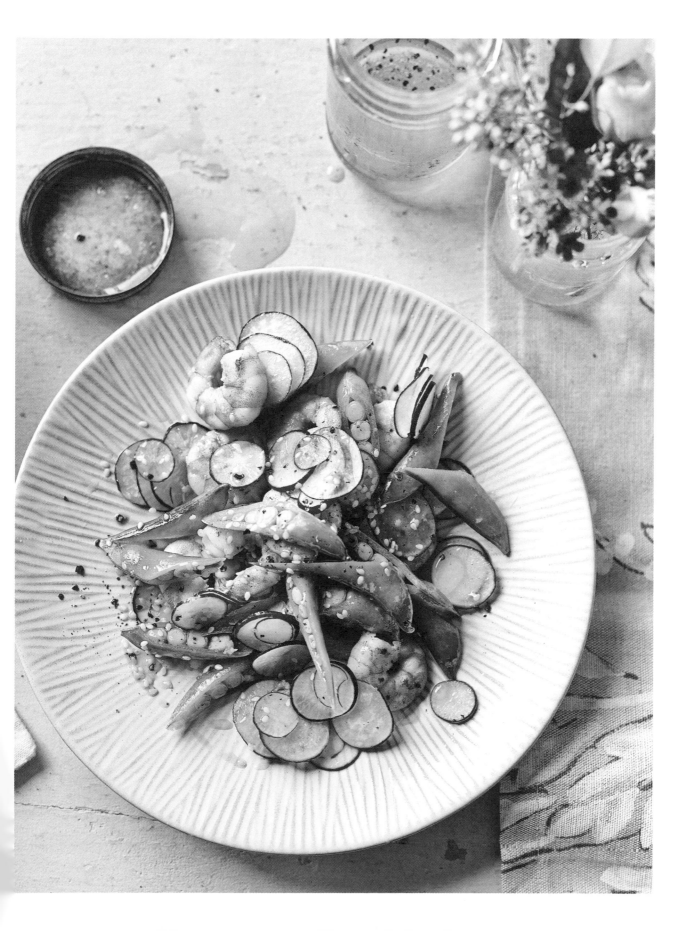

orange duck with charred chicory

Duck and orange is the ultimate combo. It sits perfectly next to the chicory, which acts as a great digestive. The figs offer some extra sweetness and look rather fancy, making this dish the ultimate date-night meal.

serves 2

1 orange
2 duck breasts
2 figs, quartered (optional; use if in season)
1 tsp coconut oil
1 head chicory, broken into individual leaves
3 tbsp chopped walnuts
2 tbsp olive oil
salt and pepper

Zest the orange and rub this into the duck breasts with a pinch of salt and good grind of pepper. Leave the duck breasts to marinate in the fridge for at least 2 hours and up to 12 hours, if you have time.

Heat a frying pan over a high heat and place the duck breast in, skin-side down first. Sear both sides for 2 minutes, then turn the heat down to medium and cook for another 10 minutes, flipping the breasts over every few minutes.

Slice the orange into 1cm slices and the figs into quarters.

Heat a griddle pan with the coconut oil. Char the chicory leaves on both sides. Serve the duck with the sliced orange, charred chicory, figs and walnuts, and drizzle over the olive oil.

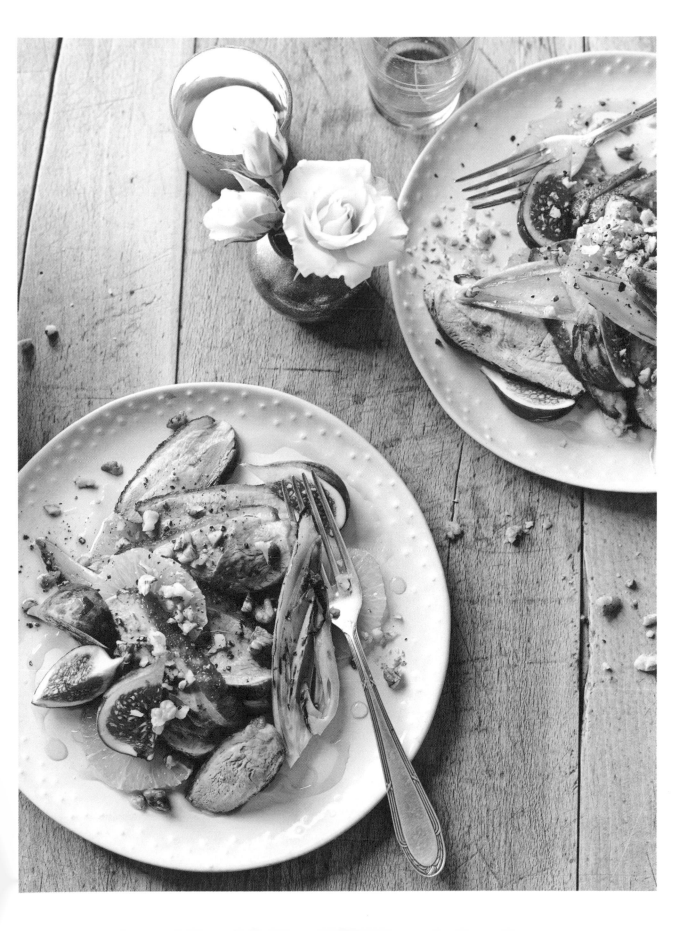

pan-fried ocean trout with a beetroot and pear salad

Here succulent trout is married with the earthy depth of beetroot and light undertones of pear. Acidity and balance are the keys to this crowd-pleaser. Walnuts give the omega-3-packed texture one longs for in such a dish.

serves 2

1 tsp mustard
2 tbsp olive oil
1 beetroot
1 fennel bulb
1 pear
10g fresh mint leaves
3 tbsp chopped walnuts
2 ocean trout fillets
1 tbsp coconut oil
salt and pepper

Whisk the mustard and olive oil together and season with salt and pepper.

Grate the beetroot, thinly slice the fennel and pear. Layer the fruit and veg with the chopped mint, walnuts and the olive oil dressing.

Heat a frying pan over a medium to high heat with the coconut oil. When the oil starts to bubble, place the trout fillets in skin-side down. Cook for 2 minutes, then flip and cook the other side for 1 minute.

Serve all the components together.

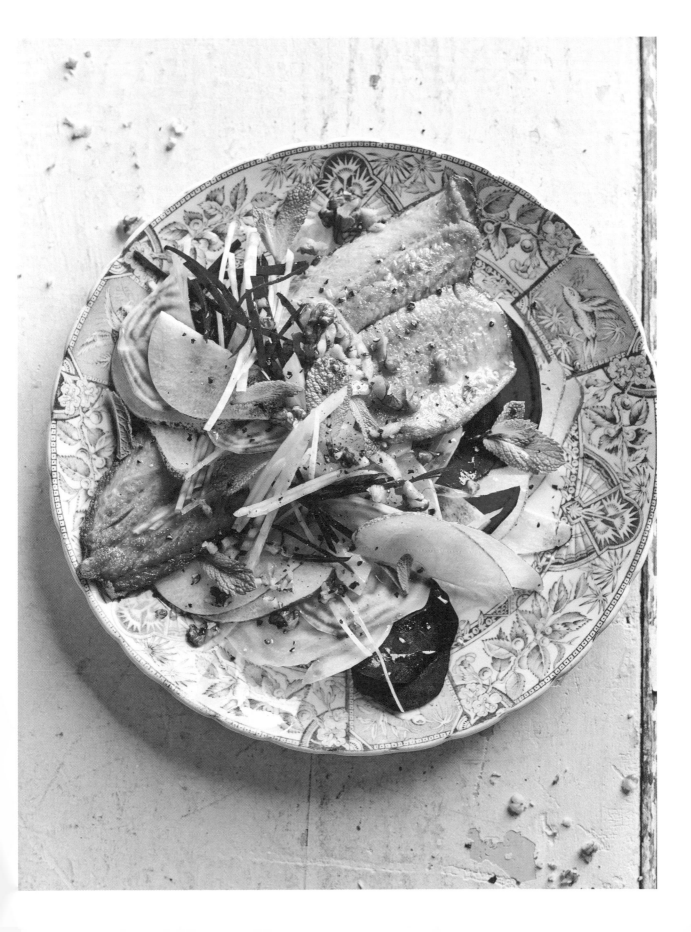

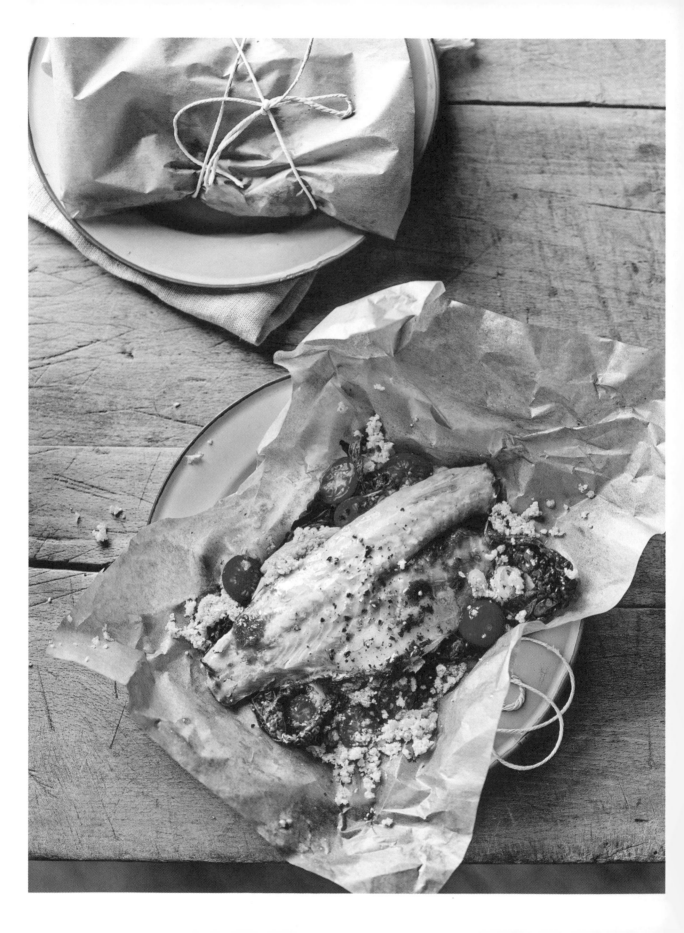

ginger steamed snapper parcel with cauliflower rice and chard

What I love most about this is its versatility. You can choose whether you want the fish or the vegetables to be the main event, and either way you won't be disappointed. Ginger and soy give an oriental aroma to this wonderful dish.

Preheat the oven to 200°C/400°F/Gas mark 6.

Rub the fish in the ginger and tamari, soy sauce or Liquid Aminos.

Put the roughly chopped cauliflower into a food processor and process for a few minutes until you have a rice-like consistency. Heat 1 tablespoon coconut oil in a pan over a medium heat. Toss the spring onions into the pan with a pinch of salt, stir-fry for a few minutes, then add the turmeric and cauliflower rice. Stir-fry for 1 minute, until the cauliflower has coloured, then take it off the heat.

Grab some foil or baking paper and cut two rectangles measuring at least 45cm in length. For each person, dollop 1 teaspoon coconut oil in the middle, then add the chard, cauliflower rice and tomatoes. Finally, place the fish on top. Grind some salt and pepper over the fish and squeeze the juice of 1 lime into each parcel. Wrap the foil or baking paper around the food and seal up the edges.

Bake for 15–20 minutes, until the fish is cooked through, and serve in the parcels.

serves 2

2 snapper fillets (or sea bass, salmon or cod)
1 tbsp freshly grated ginger
1 tbsp gluten-free tamari, soy sauce or Liquid Aminos
½ cauliflower, stalk removed and roughly chopped
1 tbsp coconut oil, plus 2 tsp
3 spring onions, chopped into ½cm pieces
1 tsp turmeric
50g Swiss chard, chopped (or any other chard or pak choi)
10 cherry tomatoes, halved
2 limes
salt and pepper

beef stir-fry with courgette noodles

serves 2

2 sirloin steaks, or another favourite cut, sliced into 2.5cm strips
2 courgettes, ends cut off
1 tbsp coconut oil
1 red onion, finely chopped
2 cloves garlic, crushed
2 tbsp freshly grated ginger
1 red chilli, finely chopped
100g sugarsnap peas, cut in half
juice of 1 lime
2 tbsp sesame seeds
1 tbsp gluten-free tamari, soy sauce or Liquid Aminos
salt and pepper

Everyone loves a stir-fry. But everyone also always asks me 'how can I make it healthier?' If you have an intolerance, remove the gluten: get your spiraliser out and make courgetti! This is so delicious, and goes perfectly with the flavours of the stir-fry. And the beef and chilli go hand in hand with all the other ingredients.

Grind salt and pepper over the steaks, and set aside.

Spiralise or julienne the courgettes, or cut them into very fine strips with a peeler to make the 'courgetti'.

Heat the coconut oil in a large wok or pan. Add the onion to the pan and cook for 5 minutes with a pinch of salt. Add the garlic, ginger and chilli, and stir-fry for a further minute. Add the steak, and stir-fry for another minute, and finally throw in the sugarsnaps and courgette. Cook for 3 minutes more, stirring constantly.

Remove from the heat and squeeze over the lime juice. Serve with the sesame seeds and tamari, soy sauce or Liquid Aminos over the top.

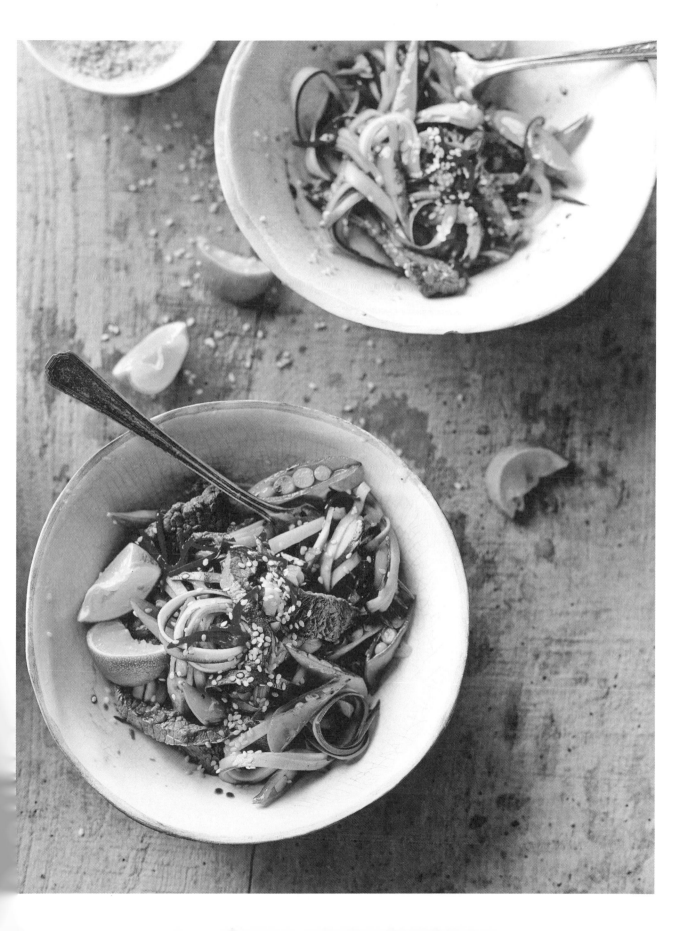

lemon sole, pancetta, peas and salsa verde

serves 2

50g flat-leaf parsley
50g basil
100ml olive oil
1 tbsp capers
1 tbsp cider vinegar
1 tsp mustard
2 lemon sole fillets
4 pancetta rashers
  (or Parma ham)
½ tbsp coconut oil
100g petits pois
zest and juice of
  1 lemon
salt and pepper

My golden rule: always make sure you have peas in the freezer. They will go in anything, and this dish illustrates that perfectly. Lemon sole is a beautiful, soft, white fish, and with the saltiness of the pancetta and that fresh burst from the peas, you have a winning combination.

Make the salsa verde first by blending the parsley, basil, olive oil, capers, vinegar and mustard in a food processor. Blend until you have a smooth paste, and set aside.

Salt and pepper the fish fillets and set them aside.

Heat a frying pan over a medium heat and grill the pancetta for 1 minute on each side, until crisp, then set aside.

Heat the same pan with the coconut oil over a medium to high heat. Wait until the oil starts to bubble, then fry the fish for 2 minutes on the first side, then 1 minute on the second. Put the cooked fish to one side.

Throw the petits pois into the pan and sauté them over a medium heat with the lemon for a few minutes, then serve to the side of the fish with a smear of salsa verde and the pancetta.

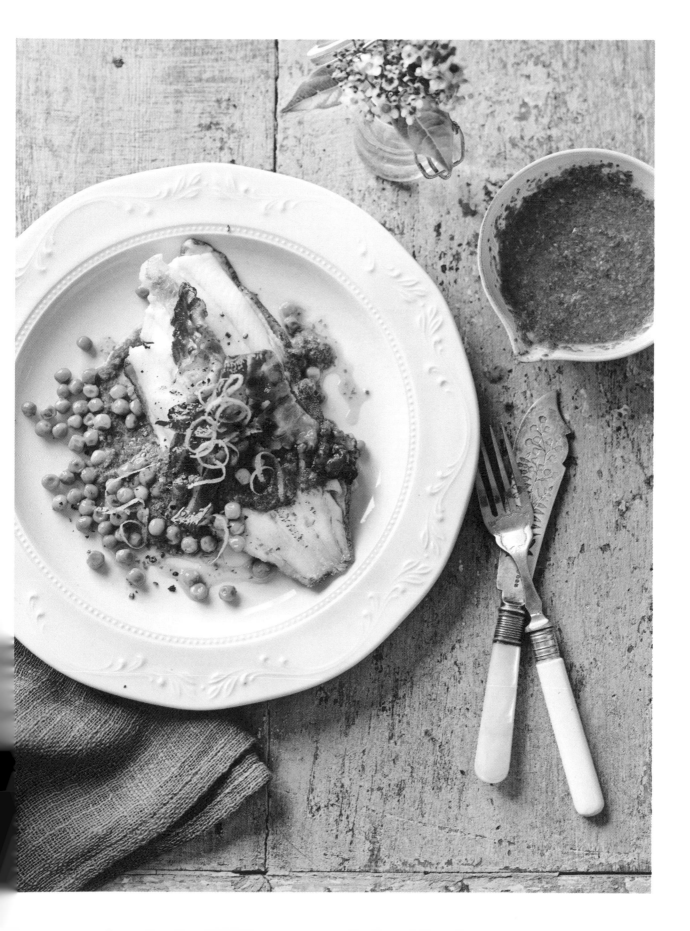

fish burgers with raw carrot slaw

serves 2

fish burger
200g haddock,
  skinned and
  roughly chopped
200g salmon,
  skinned and
  roughly chopped
1 tbsp freshly
  grated ginger
2 tsp gluten-free
  tamari, soy sauce
  or Liquid Aminos
4 tbsp chopped
  coriander
1 tbsp gluten-free
  flour (if needed)

slaw
2 large carrots,
  grated
juice of 1 lime
1 tbsp olive oil
1 tbsp freshly
  grated ginger
2 tbsp natural
  yoghurt
2 tbsp sesame
  seeds
1 tbsp coconut oil
  or butter
olive oil, for
  drizzling
salt and pepper

Fish burgers are slightly unorthodox, but so easy to make and a joy to eat! My raw slaw is super-light, using yoghurt instead of mayonnaise, and with that much-needed crunch from grated carrot, as well as sesame seeds, it's perfectly textured.

To make the burgers, whizz the chopped fish in the food processor with the rest of the burger ingredients and a grind of salt and pepper. Form the mixture into four patties on a plate, add a little gluten-free flour if the pattie mix is too moist, and refrigerate for 30 minutes.

Mix the grated carrot with the lime juice, olive oil, ginger, yoghurt, sesame seeds and a pinch of salt.

Heat a pan with the coconut oil or butter over a medium to high heat, and fry the patties for 4 minutes on each side. Serve two patties per person with the slaw and a little drizzle of olive oil.

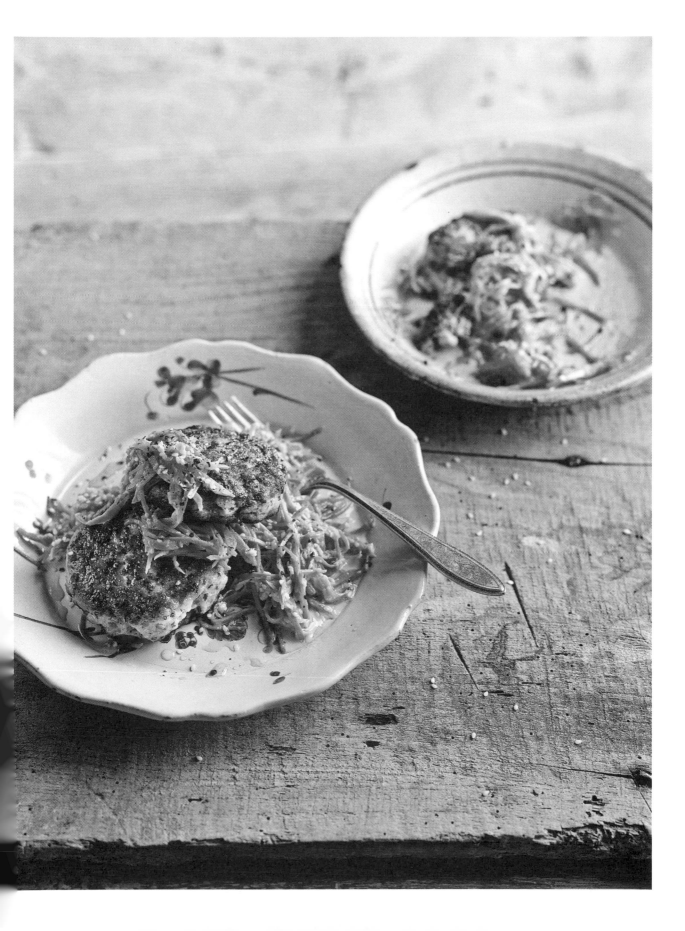

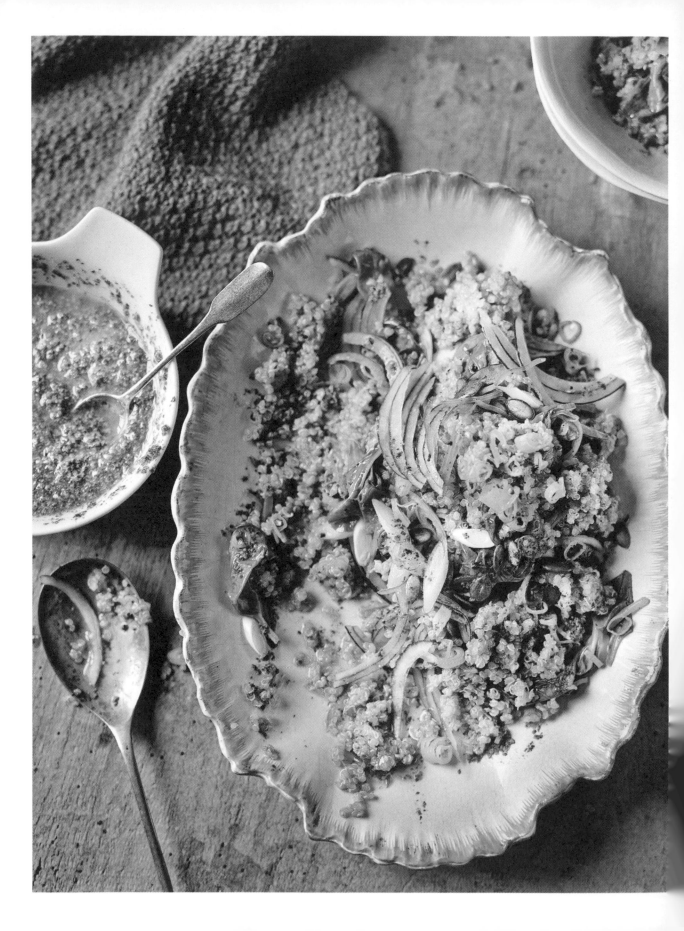

green queen quinoa dish

This ticks the boxes for both vegetarians and protein loaders. My senses were excited by the multiple textures going on here. Quinoa, onion, pumpkin seeds … all steeped in seasoned stock or water. A suggestion of fresh chopped chilli as a garnish always makes me happy.

Put the quinoa in a saucepan with the boiling water or stock and a pinch of salt. Bring it to the boil, then turn the heat down and let it gently simmer for 12–15 minutes, or until all the liquid has been absorbed.

Heat a large frying pan, and dry-roast the cumin for 1 minute. When the quinoa is cooked through, add the toasted cumin and the spinach leaves, and stir until they are fully combined and the spinach starts to wilt.

Add the red onion, spring onions, green chilli and pumpkin seeds to the quinoa mix, and pour into a serving bowl.

In a blender, blend the dressing ingredients. Slather the dressing over the quinoa.

serves 4

250g quinoa
500ml boiling
  water or chicken
  stock
1 tsp ground cumin
100g spinach
  leaves
½ red onion, finely
  sliced
3 spring onions,
  finely sliced
1 fresh green chilli,
  deseeded and
  finely chopped
50g pumpkin seeds
pinch salt

dressing
25g mint
100g basil
3 tbsp tahini
juice of 1 lime
80ml olive oil
salt and pepper

buckwheat, asparagus and pea risotto

serves 2

150g buckwheat
1 tbsp coconut oil
1 small white onion,
   finely chopped
2 cloves garlic,
   crushed
250ml chicken or
   vegetable stock
1 x 400ml can
   coconut milk
zest and juice of
   1 lemon
100g petits pois
3 spring onions,
   finely chopped
1 bunch asparagus
25g mint leaves
4 tbsp chopped
   walnuts
salt and pepper

This has all the flavours and textures of spring. The creamy coconut offers a dairy-free alternative to this familiar dish, while the protein-packed buckwheat adds a wonderfully nutty taste.

Rinse the buckwheat in a sieve. Heat a pan with the coconut oil for 1 minute over a medium heat, then throw in the onion and a pinch of salt and sauté for 5 minutes, or until the onion is lightly bronzed. Add the garlic and the buckwheat, and stir-fry for another minute. Pour in the stock, and allow to simmer for 10 minutes with a lid on.

Open the coconut milk and separate the coconut milk from the cream. (The cream is at the top and is more solid, and the milk is the liquid at the bottom. If the contents of the can are mostly solid, warm 100g of the coconut cream with 50ml water.)

Take the lid off the pan, and gradually add the lemon zest and juice, petits pois, spring onions and coconut milk. Make sure you keep stirring constantly, and cook for 10 minutes. For the last 7 minutes place the asparagus on top, and pop a lid back on the pan to let the spears steam.

Remove the asparagus spears and set aside. Stir the coconut cream into the mixture in the pan, with good grind of salt and pepper.

Scatter the mint leaves over the plated risotto with the asparagus and the chopped walnuts.

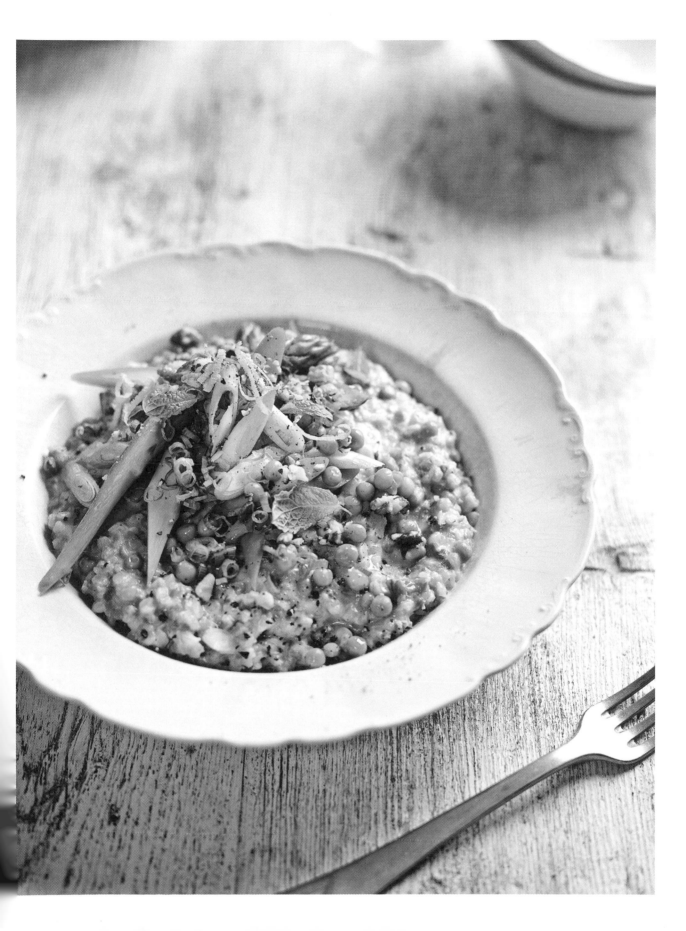

sesame seared tuna salad, pea mash and bean shoots

serves 2

6 tbsp sesame
  seeds, toasted
2 tuna steaks
2 tbsp gluten-free
  tamari, soy sauce
  or Liquid Aminos
1 large clove garlic,
  crushed
1 tbsp honey
4 tsp coconut oil
1 shallot, finely
  diced
300g frozen petits
  pois
2 limes
2 tsp freshly grated
  ginger
1 tbsp tahini
50g beansprouts
fresh coriander
  leaves, to serve
salt and pepper

This simple dish can be whipped up in minutes. I like to keep the tuna steak rare and slice it thin. The tahini sauce gives the dish a gingery finish and ups your calcium intake for the day.

Spread the sesame seeds on a plate. Rub the tuna steaks in the tamari, soy sauce or Liquid Aminos and the crushed garlic and honey, then put them in the sesame seeds to coat both sides.

Heat 1 teaspoon coconut oil in a large frying pan over a medium heat, then throw in the shallot with a pinch of salt, and cook for 5 minutes. Next add the petits pois, 2 tablespoons water, ground pepper and the juice of 1 lime, and cook for 4 minutes. Blend the pan mixture in a blender until puréed.

Heat a frying pan over a high heat with the remaining coconut oil. Wait until it is hot, then sear the tuna steaks for 2 minutes one side then for 1½ minutes on the other side; this will keep it pink in the middle.

Mix the ginger, tahini and zest and juice of 1 lime together. Plate the tuna, beansprouts and pea purée on two plates and slather with the dressing. Serve with fresh coriander.

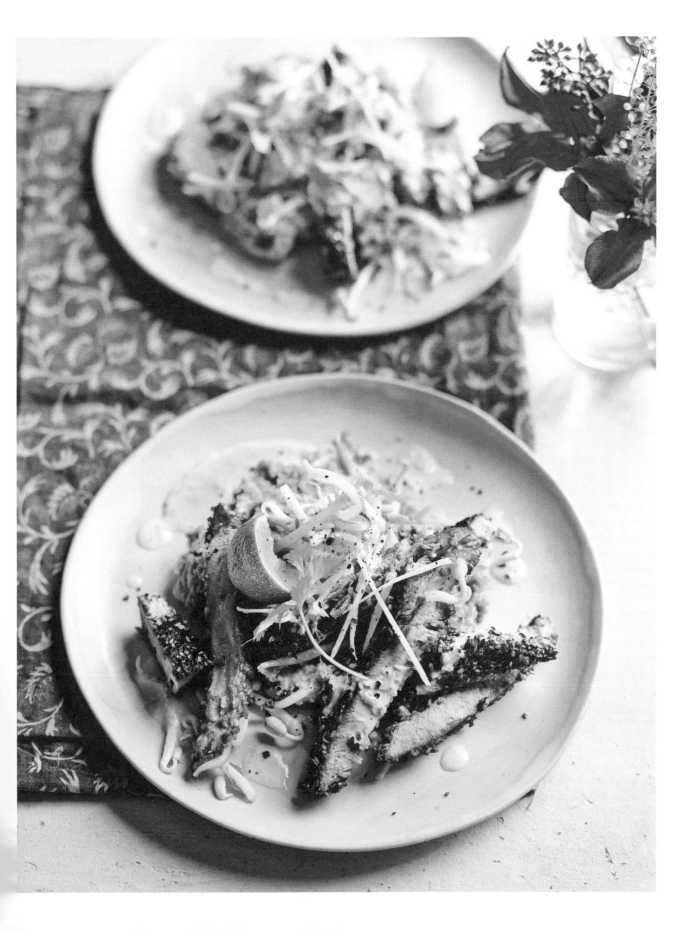

monkfish curry with indian spiced cauliflower rice

serves 4
400g monkfish, cut
  into bite-size chunks
2 tsp turmeric
3 tbsp fresh grated
  ginger
1 tbsp coconut oil or
  butter
1 white onion, finely
  sliced
1 red chilli, deseeded
  and finely chopped
1 clove garlic, crushed
1 x 400ml can coconut
  milk
juice of 1 lime
1 tbsp mustard seeds
1 handful fresh
  coriander, finely
  chopped
salt and pepper

Indian spiced
cauliflower rice
1 cauliflower, stalk
  removed and
  roughly chopped
1 tbsp coconut oil or
  butter
1 tsp turmeric
½ tsp ground cumin
¼ tsp cinnamon
¼ tsp ground ginger
fresh coriander,
  to serve

I actually made this dish up trying to impress my boyfriend, whose family is Indian. I think it worked.

Put the chunks of fish in a bowl with a pinch of salt, the turmeric and the ginger. Massage the spices into the fillets and marinate.

Heat the coconut oil or butter in a large pan over a medium heat. Add the onions and a pinch of salt, and sauté for 5 minutes.

Add the chilli and garlic. Stir-fry for a minute, then add the coconut milk, lime juice and some freshly ground pepper, and let this all simmer for 5 minutes. Finally, throw in the fish and simmer gently for 10 minutes, or until the fish is cooked through. Remove from the heat.

In a small frying pan, dry-roast the mustard seeds for 1 minute, then crush them slightly.

Sprinkle the fresh coriander and mustard seeds over the top of the curry, and serve with Indian Spiced Cauliflower Rice, below.

indian spiced cauliflower rice

Put the roughly chopped cauliflower into a food processor and process for a few minutes until you get a rice-like consistency.

Heat the coconut oil or butter in a pan over a medium heat for 1 minute, then add the spices and stir for 1 minute more until fragrant.

Add the cauliflower 'rice' and sauté for 3 minutes, stirring constantly, until cooked through. Serve sprinkled with some fresh coriander.

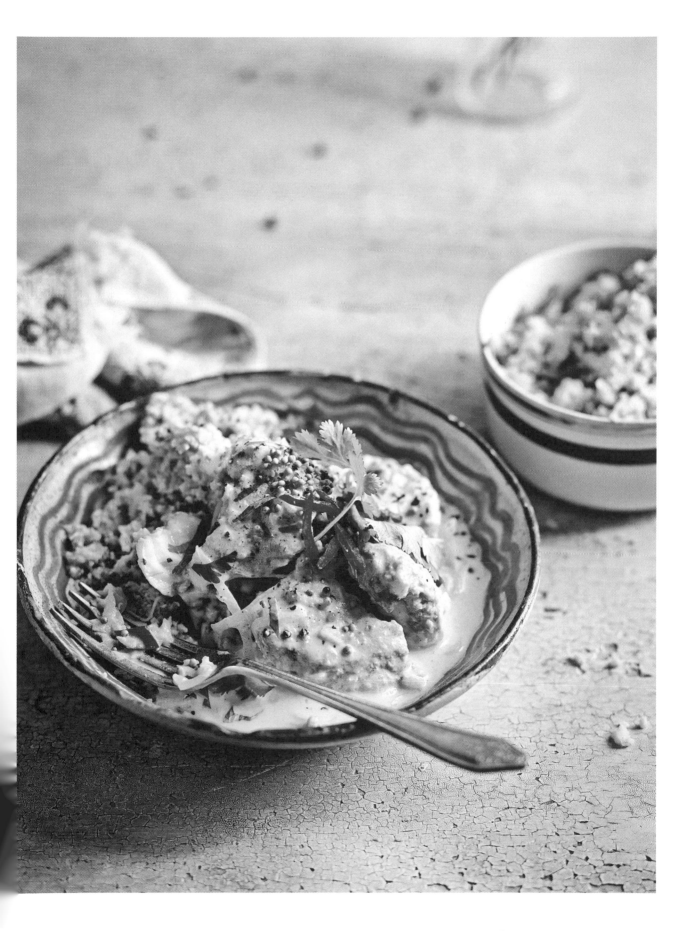

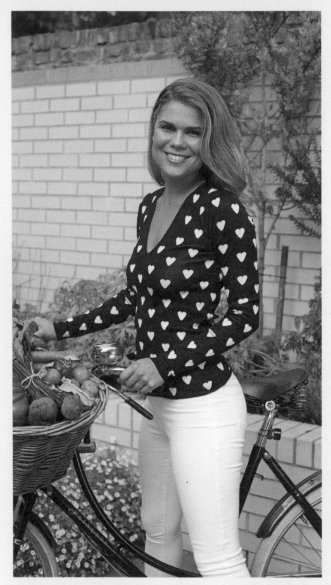

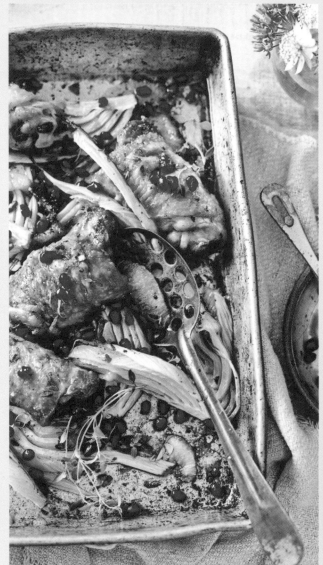

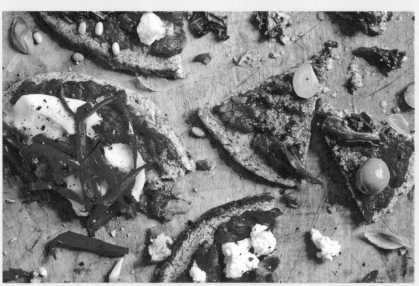

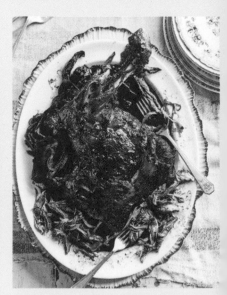

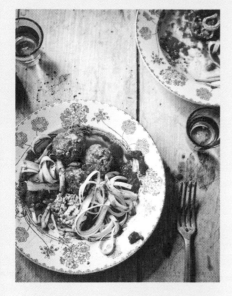

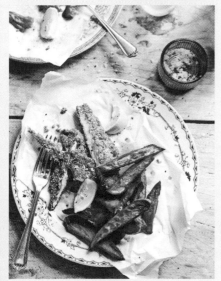

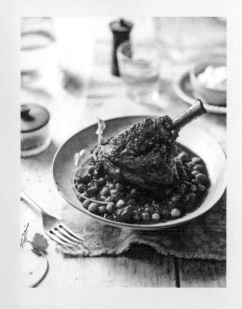

weekend wonders

smoky roast chicken with sweet potato wedges

This is the gift that keeps on giving. Make it on Sunday, and enjoy it throughout the week. Sweet potato offers a lower-starch alternative to regular potato varieties, and when you have an organic, free-range roast chicken in the fridge, no one will complain.

serves 6

6 tbsp coconut oil
2 tbsp cayenne pepper
2 tbsp smoked paprika
zest and juice of 1 lime
1.5kg whole chicken
5 sweet potatoes, cut into wedges
4 cloves garlic, crushed
salt and pepper

Preheat the oven to 200°C/400°F/Gas mark 6.

In a frying pan melt the coconut oil with the spices, garlic and lime zest and juice over a very low heat. Rub the spicy oil all over the chicken and sweet potato wedges, massaging every part of the chicken. Grind a generous amount of salt and pepper over both. Put the chicken in a large roasting tin and roast for 1 hour 20 minutes. After 35 minutes scatter the sweet potato wedges around the outside of the chicken and let them cook with the chicken for the last 45 minutes.

Let the cooked chicken rest for 5 minutes, and serve with the sweet potato wedges.

Once cooked this will keep in the fridge all week, and can be used for lunches.

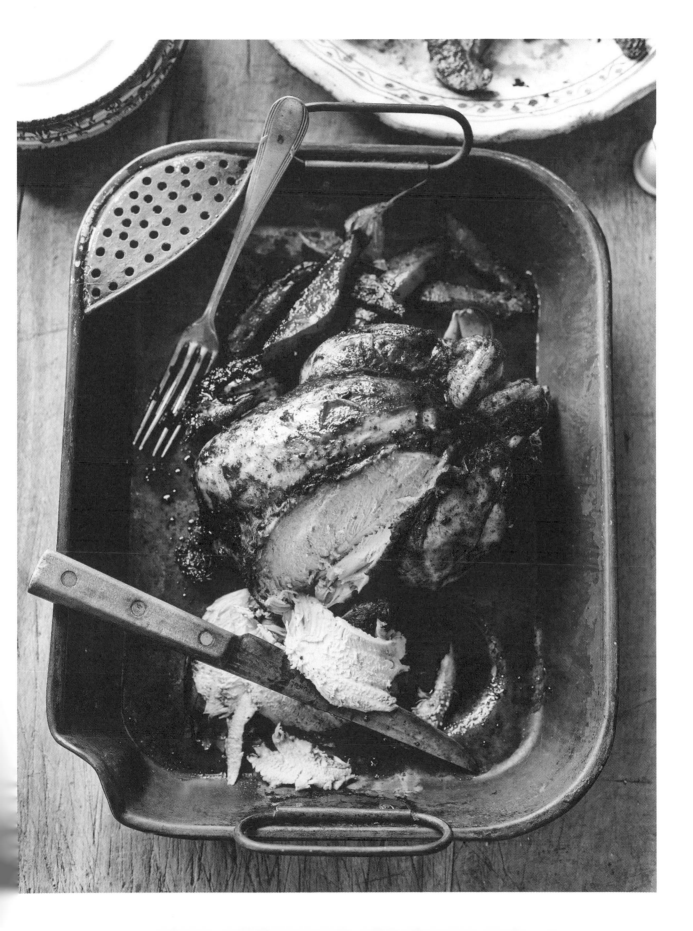

slow-roast lamb shank

serves 2

2 tbsp coconut oil
  or butter
2 tsp paprika
1 white onion,
  finely sliced
pinch salt
1 red chilli, finely
  sliced
1 x 400g can
  chickpeas,
  drained
1 x 400g can
  tomatoes
3 tbsp tomato
  purée
2 sprigs thyme
2 lamb shanks

fresh coriander and
  natural yoghurt,
  to serve

I like my meat to fall off the bone. Not only does it taste better, it is also nutritionally better to cook meat at a lower temperature. Serve this up on a cold night – it's a crowd-pleaser.

Set your slow cooker to low, or preheat the oven to 130°C/250°F/ Gas mark ½.

Heat 1 tablespoon coconut oil or butter in a large pot for 1 minute with the paprika, over a medium to high heat. Add the onion along with a pinch of salt, and sauté for 5 minutes. Add the chilli and cook for a further minute. Toss the drained chickpeas in and cook, stirring, for another minute. Add the tomatoes, tomato purée and thyme, and let everything cook for 5 minutes more.

In a large frying pan, heat the remaining tablespoon of coconut oil or butter for 1 minute over a high heat. Add the lamb shanks, and brown them all over for 1 minute, then throw them into the tomato and chickpea mixture.

If slow cooking – put everything in the slow cooker for 4 hours. If cooking in the oven – put the pot in the oven with the lid on for 4 hours.

The meat should fall off the bone when it is ready. Serve with fresh coriander and dollops of yoghurt.

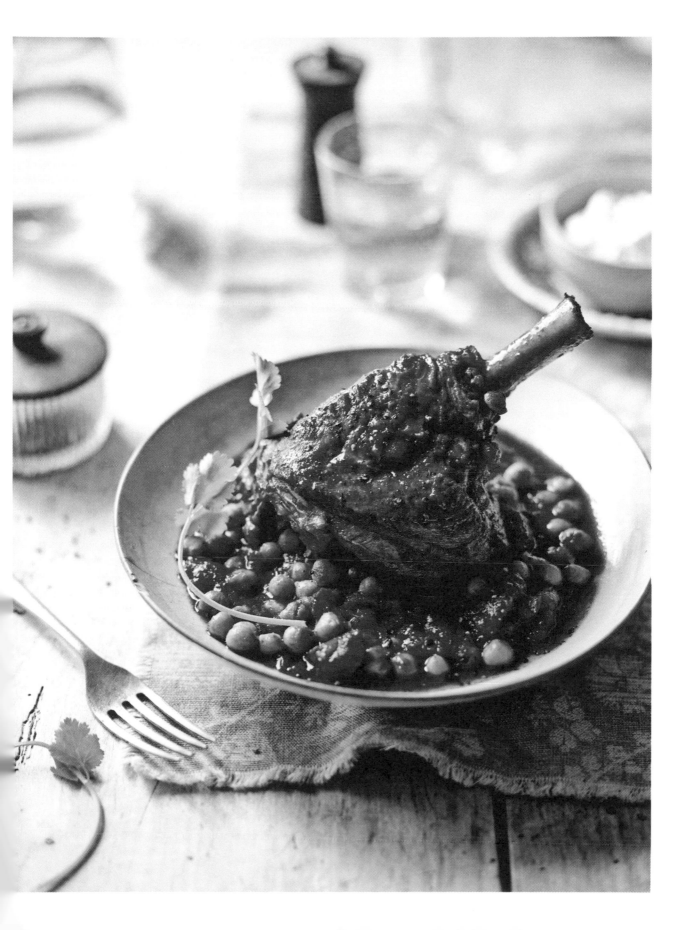

beef stew with apricots

I adore beef. It absorbs flavours so well, and the key to it (in my opinion) is to cook it slowly. Whatever you don't eat can be frozen, to be enjoyed later. Apricots bring a wonderful sweetness, and here you also get all the antioxidant benefits of cumin.

serves 4

500g organic stewing beef
1 tbsp ground cumin
1 tsp paprika
1 large white onion, chopped
2 tbsp coconut oil or butter
1 red pepper, chopped into small chunks
100g dried apricots
1 x 400g can chopped tomatoes
3 tbsp tomato purée
salt and pepper

Rub the meat with the cumin, paprika and a pinch of salt and pepper.

In a large frying pan, brown the onions in 1 tablespoon coconut oil or butter. Add the pepper to the pan with the apricots, chopped tomatoes and tomato purée.

Heat the remaining 1 tablespoon coconut oil or butter in another pan, and brown the meat on all sides for 1 minute. Add the browned meat to the pepper, apricots and tomatoes, and stir. Leave to simmer over a low heat for 2 hours.

This works well served with Classic Plain Cauliflower Rice (see page 210).

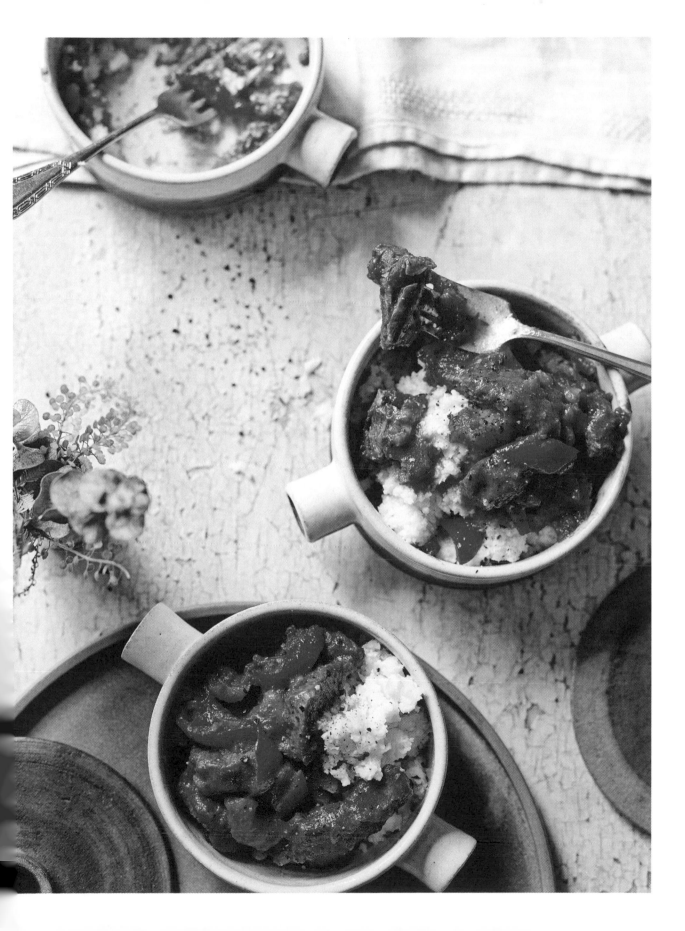

chickpea and lentil dhal with coconut cauliflower rice

serves 4

1 tsp turmeric
1 tsp chilli powder
2 tsp ground cumin
1 tbsp coconut oil
1 red onion,
  roughly chopped
2 cloves garlic
3cm freshly grated
  ginger
1 x 400ml can
  coconut milk
1 x 400g can
  chickpeas,
  drained
150g dried red
  lentils
100g spinach
  leaves
salt and pepper

coconut cauliflower rice
serves 4

1 cauliflower, stalk
  removed and
  roughly chopped
1 tbsp coconut oil
1 white onion,
  finely diced
½ tsp ground
  cardamom
200ml coconut
  milk

The combined flavours in this dish make for an incomparable taste sensation. It may be vegetarian, but it offers a solid source of protein in the form of lentils. It is best enjoyed on a cold evening, snuggled up with a movie.

Put the dry spices in a frying pan, and dry-fry for 1 minute with a pinch of salt. Heat the coconut oil over a medium heat for 1 minute, then add the onion and sauté for 5 minutes. Add the garlic and ginger and stir-fry for a few minutes more, then pour in the coconut milk with a pinch of salt and a good grind of pepper. Add the drained chickpeas and the lentils. Cook, covered, for 40 minutes. For the last 5 minutes, drop in the spinach and stir so it wilts in with the mix.

Serve with the Coconut Cauliflower Rice, below.

coconut cauliflower rice

Put the roughly chopped cauliflower into a food processor and process for a few minutes until you get a rice-like consistency.

Heat the coconut oil in a large pot over a medium to high heat, then add the onion and cook for 5 minutes. Throw in the cardamom and stir for 30 seconds, then add the cauliflower 'rice' and coconut milk, and cook for a further 10 minutes.

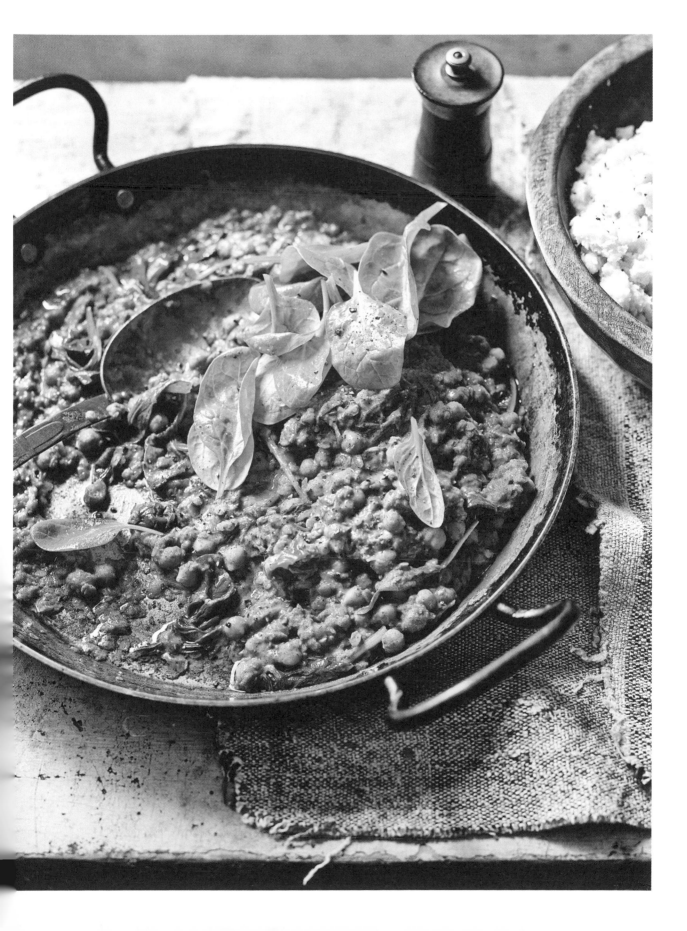

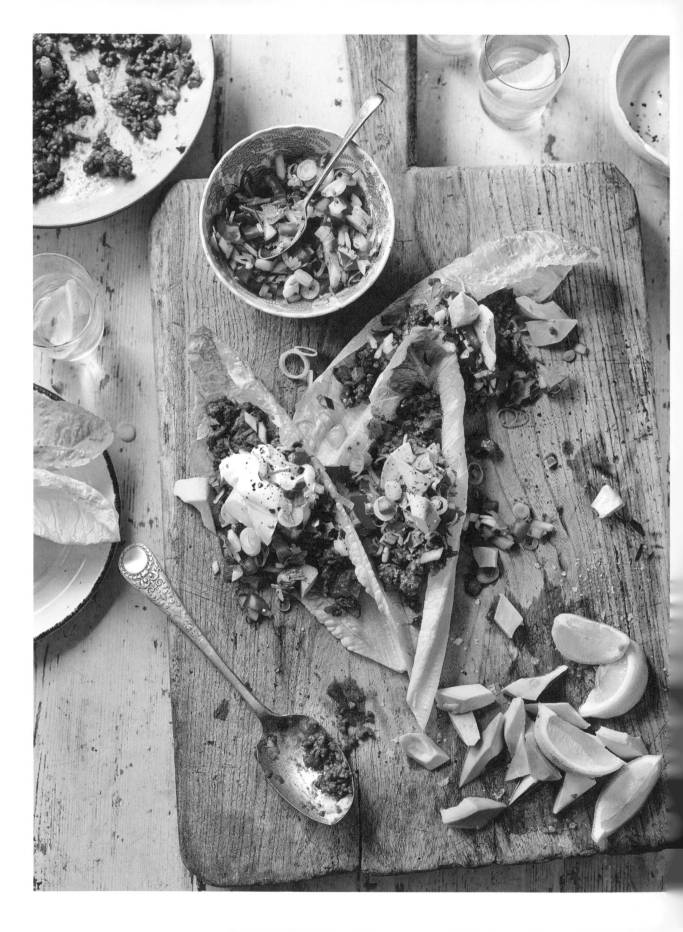

mexican mince in lettuce wraps with fresh salsa

This is one of my signature dishes, and for me it's all about sharing. Everyone can get stuck in with this multi-faceted approach to a Mexican classic. I take a lettuce leaf, load it with hearty spiced meat, soften it with avocado … and never forget the salsa kick. Perfect.

In a large frying pan, dry-roast the cumin, paprika and chilli for 1 minute over a medium heat, then turn the heat down a little and add the coconut oil, celery, onion and a pinch of salt. Sauté over a medium heat for 5 minutes. Add the mince, stirring with a spoon and allowing it to bronze for 1 minute. Pour in the tomatoes. Let it all gently simmer for 1 hour, stirring regularly. This can be made the day before and reheated (it gets better with age).

To make the salsa, mix all the ingredients in a bowl.

Cut the avocados into cubes, and sprinkle over a pinch of salt and the lemon juice.

When the mince is ready, juice the lime into it and give it a stir. Serve with the lettuce leaves as wraps, along with the avocado, yoghurt and salsa.

serves 4

mexican mince
1 tsp ground cumin
1 tsp paprika
1 tsp chilli powder
1 tbsp coconut oil
2 sticks celery, finely chopped
1 white onion, finely chopped
500g beef or lamb mince
1 x 400g can tomatoes
1 lime

salsa
2 spring onions, chopped into small cubes
3 tomatoes, chopped into small cubes
1 cucumber, chopped into small cubes
1 red chilli, deseeded and finely diced
juice of 1 lime
2 tbsp chopped fresh coriander
2 avocados, peeled and cut into chunks
1 lemon, cut into wedges
1 large cos lettuce, leaves separated
100g natural yoghurt
salt and pepper

squash curry with ginger and lime rice

serves 3–4

50g fresh coriander
2 tbsp red curry
    paste
1 x 400ml can
    coconut milk
1 tbsp tomato pureé
½ tsp turmeric
1 tbsp coconut oil
1 white onion,
    finely chopped
pinch salt
400g butternut
    squash or
    pumpkin, peeled
    and cubed
150g green beans,
    ends cut off
50g spinach leaves
juice of 1 lime

ginger and lime rice
1 cauliflower, stalk
    removed and
    roughly chopped
1 tbsp coconut oil
zest and juice of
    1 lime
1 tbsp fresh grated
    ginger
2 tbsp chopped
    fresh coriander
3 tbsp water

I love squash. It's tasty, filling and absorbs other flavours amazingly. Meanwhile, spinach provides an abundance of iron and a bit of colour for those who like to make their dishes look pretty. I certainly do.

Separate the coriander leaves from the stalks. Set aside the leaves for the final garnish and finely chop the stalks.

In a food processor or blender, blitz the coriander stalks, red curry paste, coconut milk, tomato purée and turmeric.

Heat the coconut oil in a pan over a medium heat for 1 minute. Put the onions into the pan. Sauté them for 5 minutes with a pinch of salt. Add the squash and stir-fry for 1 minute, then pour in the blended mix, bring to a simmer and let this cook for 10 minutes. Add the green beans and spinach and cook for another 20 minutes until the pumpkin is cooked through.

Meanwhile, make the Ginger and Lime Rice. Put the roughly chopped cauliflower into a food processor and process for a few minutes until you get a rice-like consistency.

Heat the coconut oil in a large frying pan, and throw in the lime zest with the ginger and coriander. Stir for 30 seconds, then add the cauliflower, the water and the juice of the lime. Cook for 5 minutes, until cooked through.

Scatter the coriander leaves over the curry with a squeeze of fresh lime juice, and serve with the 'rice'.

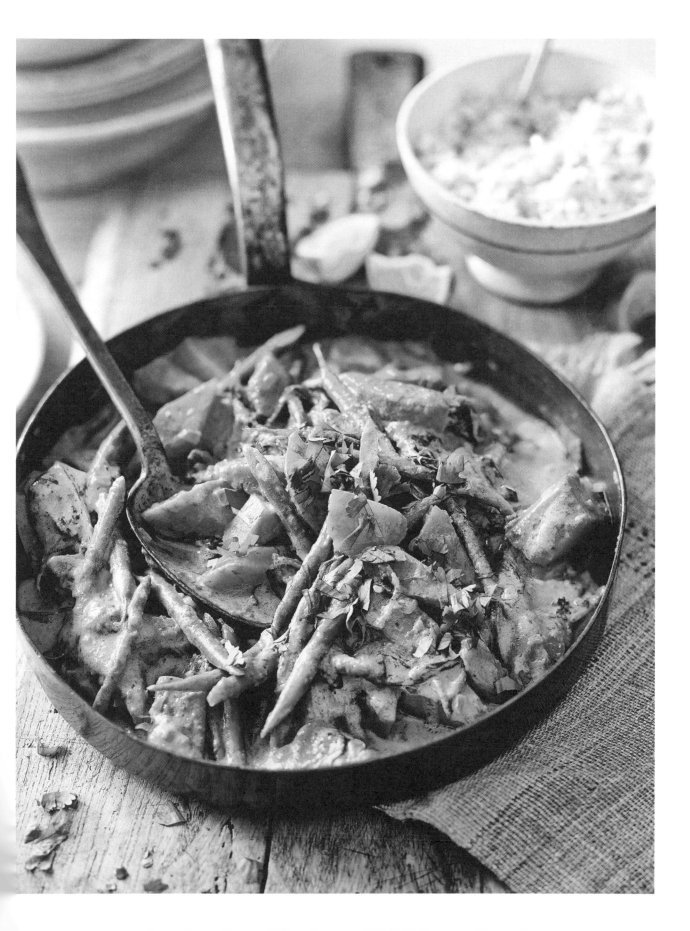

tomato turkey meatballs with homemade tomato sauce and courgetti

serves 4

600g turkey mince
1 white onion, very finely diced
3 cloves garlic
10g fresh coriander, chopped
1 tsp paprika
2 eggs, beaten
1 tbsp coconut oil
2 sticks celery, very finely diced
2 tsp chopped fresh rosemary
2 x 400g cans tomatoes
4 courgettes, ends cut off
salt and pepper

We don't eat turkey enough, as people tend to associate it with Christmas. But it's so lean, and when done properly it's beyond delicious. When teamed with my classic 'courgetti' (the best alternative to pasta, helping you avoid the bloat!) and a hearty homemade tomato sauce, I think even the Italians would love this.

Preheat the oven to 180°C/350°F/Gas mark 4.

Put the mince, half of the onion, 2 crushed garlic cloves, the coriander, the paprika and eggs into a bowl. Combine with your hands, and grind in some salt and pepper. Roll the mixture into 3cm balls and set aside in the fridge.

Heat the coconut oil in a saucepan over a medium heat for 1 minute, then add the rest of the onion, the rest of the crushed garlic and the celery, and sauté with a pinch of salt for 5 minutes. Add the rosemary and continue to cook, stirring, for 1 minute. Add the tomatoes, a pinch of salt and some ground pepper, and simmer for 10 minutes.

Meanwhile, spiralise or julienne the courgettes, or cut them into very fine strips with a peeler to make the 'courgetti'.

Take the meatballs out of the fridge. Put them in a roasting tin, and pour over the tomato sauce. Bake in the oven for 20 minutes. Serve with the courgetti.

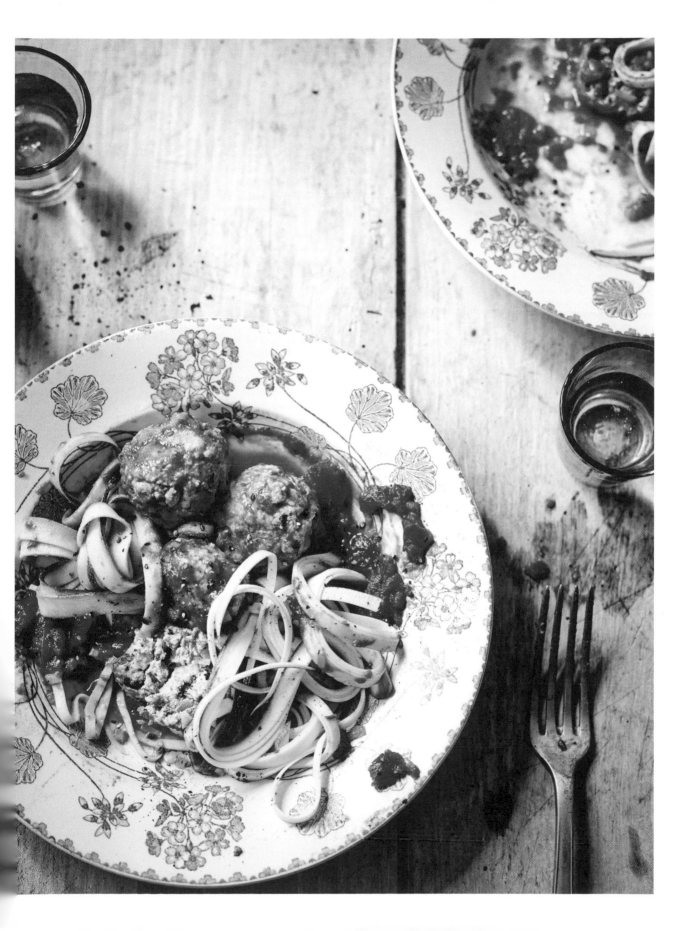

orange, fennel and pomegranate chicken

Every element of this dish contributes to making it easy to eat, easy to digest and – most importantly – easy to enjoy. Fennel is great for the stomach, and the antioxidants you get from pomegranate give the chicken a perfect finish.

serves 2

1 orange
4 tbsp coconut oil or melted butter
1 tbsp thyme
2 tsp sea salt
1 tsp freshly ground black pepper
4 chicken thighs
2 small fennel bulbs, quartered
½ a pomegranate

Preheat the oven to 200°C/400°F/Gas mark 6.

Zest the orange, and cut it into eighths. Put the orange zest, coconut oil or butter, thyme, salt and pepper in a bowl. Massage the chicken with this marinade, then put the fennel and orange pieces in too, and mix them with the marinade – try not to break the fennel up.

Place the chicken in a roasting tin, skin facing up, with the fennel and orange pieces in between. Roast for 45 minutes. Halfway through the roasting time, take the chicken out and baste it with the juices from the tin.

Bash out the pomegranate seeds with a spoon, then remove the white pith and sprinkle them over the top of the roasted chicken to serve.

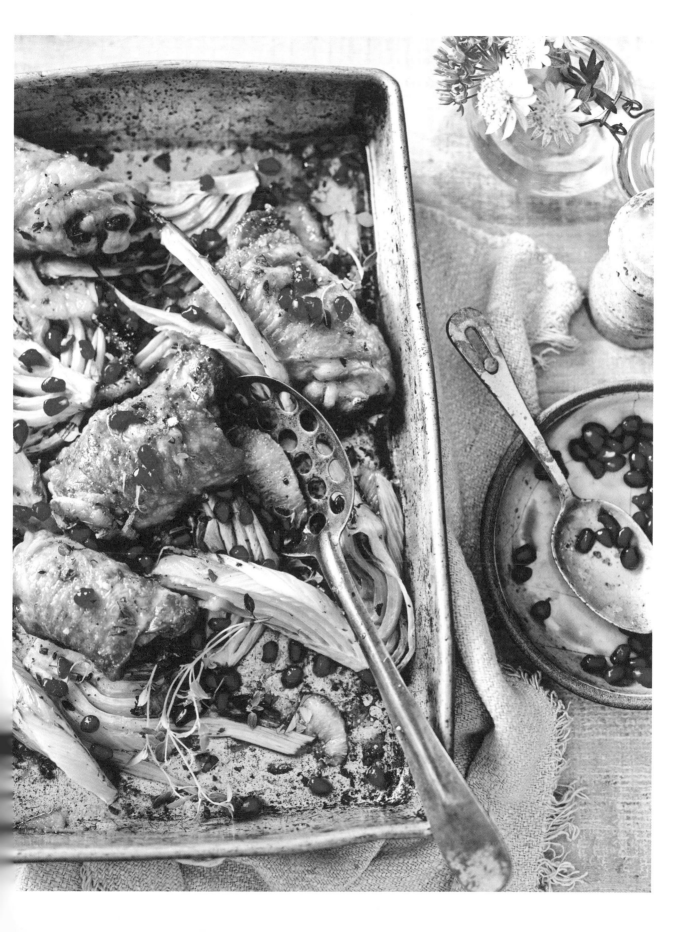

cauliflower pizza four ways

**makes 2 pizza bases
with tomato sauce**

basic base
1 small cauliflower,
stalk removed and
roughly chopped
2 egg whites,
whisked
1 tbsp oregano
6 tbsp quinoa
flour (or other
gluten-free flour
alternative)
1 tsp coconut oil,
melted
1 tbsp coconut oil
1 white onion, very
finely chopped
1 tsp dried
rosemary
1 x 400g can
tomatoes
salt

Quite simply: the best invention ever. Gluten-free, fun to make and delicious. I like to mix up my toppings, so I've given you a few ways to enjoy your pizza feast. The base is always the same, and the garnishes are up to you.

Preheat the oven to 180°C/350°F/Gas mark 4.

Put the cauliflower into the food processor and pulse until you have a fine texture (smaller than rice, but not quite flour). Add the egg whites, a large pinch of salt, the oregano and the flour, and blitz until a dough forms.

Grab a baking sheet, line it with baking paper and put half of the dough on it. Place another square of baking paper over the top, then roll or press out the pizza base with a rolling pin or spoon, until you have a circle about 1cm thick. Repeat with the other half of the dough on a separate baking sheet.

Brush the melted coconut oil over the pizza bases. Put them both in the oven and cook for 20 minutes.

Meanwhile, heat the tablespoon of coconut oil in a saucepan over a medium heat for 1 minute, then add the onion, rosemary and a pinch of salt and sauté for 5 minutes. Add the tomatoes and cook for another 10 minutes at a medium simmer until the sauce is slightly reduced.

Pour the tomato mix on top of the base, and get ready to add your choice of toppings . . .

bacon and ricotta

200g ricotta, cut into chunks
6 bacon rashers, cut into bite-size chunks

Put the cheese and bacon on after the tomato sauce, and cook at 180°C/350°F/Gas mark 4 for 8–10 minutes.

pesto, sun-dried tomato and green olives

3 tbsp Homemade Pesto (see page 72)
50g sun-dried tomatoes
50g green olives

Cook the pizza with the tomato sauce on it for 8–10 minutes at 180°C/350°F/Gas mark 4. Sprinkle on the toppings after the pizza is cooked.

cheese and pepper

½ red pepper, sliced into 1cm strips
100g mozzarella, thinly sliced
1 red chilli, deseeded and finely chopped

Put all the ingredients on after the tomato sauce, and cook at 180°C/350°F/Gas mark 4 for 8–10 minutes.

goat's cheese, spinach and pine nuts

100g spinach leaves
100g goat's cheese, torn into chunks
50g pine nuts
salt and pepper

Boil some water and soak the spinach in it for a minute, then drain. Put all the ingredients on after the tomato sauce, and cook at 180°C/350°F/Gas mark 4 for 8–10 minutes.

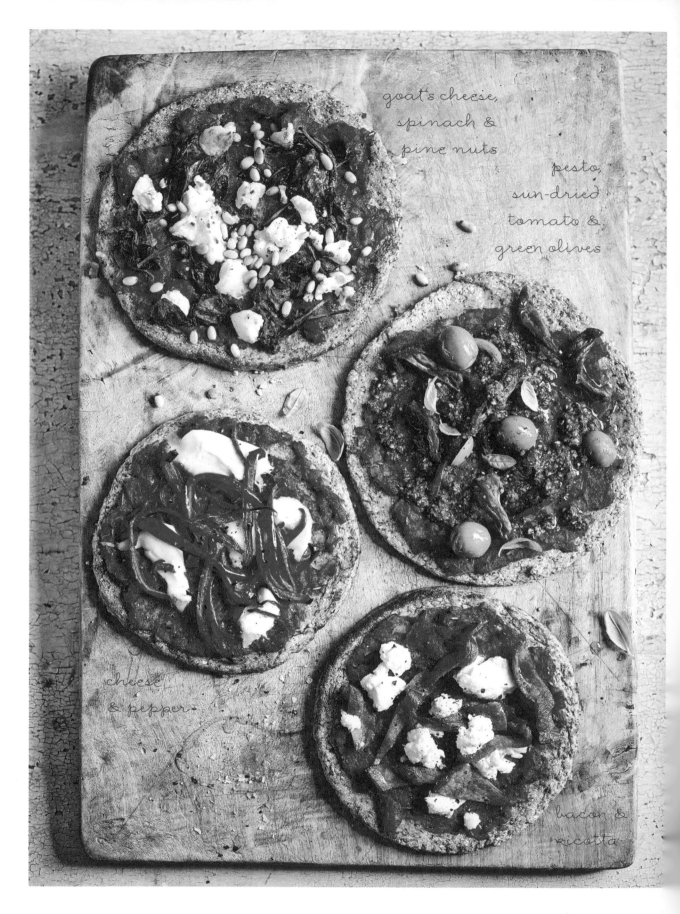

goat's cheese,
spinach &
pine nuts

pesto,
sun-dried
tomato &
green olives

cheese
& pepper

bacon &
ricotta

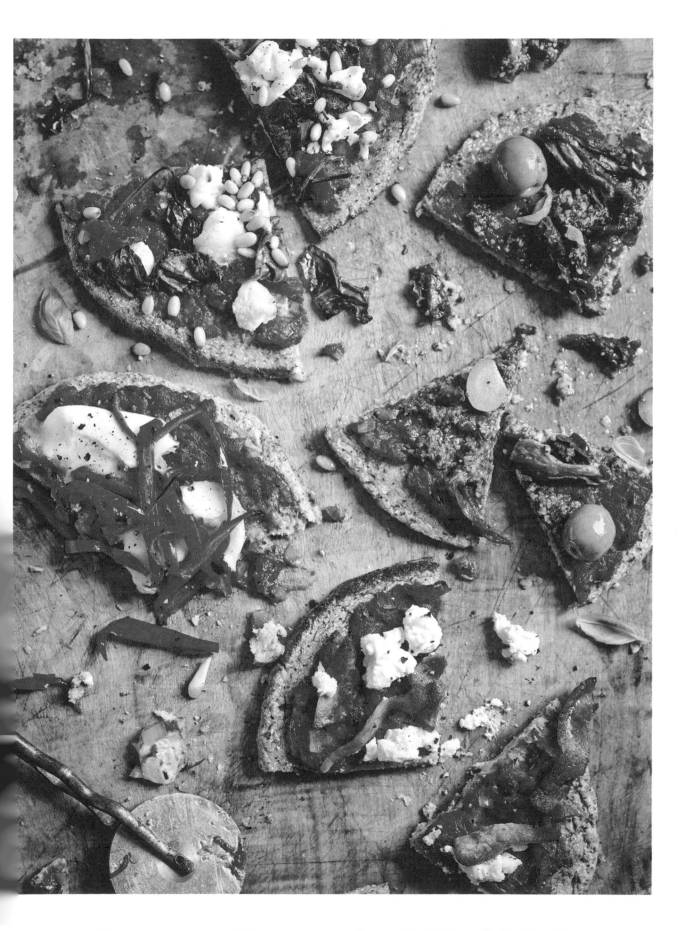

quinoa burgers with tahini sauce

serves 2 (makes 6 patties)

125g quinoa
250ml boiling water
  or chicken stock
1 courgette, grated
2 spring onions,
  finely chopped
2 cloves garlic,
  crushed
2 eggs, beaten
zest of 1 lime
30g chives, chopped
30g quinoa flour (or
  ground almonds,
  buckwheat flour, oat
  flour or rice flour)
salt and pepper

tahini sauce
1 clove garlic, crushed
50g tahini
1 tsp ground cumin
juice of 1 lime
1 tsp miso paste
1 tbsp olive oil
1 tbsp coconut oil

1 small cos lettuce,
  leaves separated,
  to serve

While I am a meat lover, it's nice to have a veggie burger once in a while. I adore this sweet tahini sauce, and it complements the gluten-free bun alternative wonderfully. Perfect for the barbecue!

Put the quinoa in a saucepan with the boiling water or stock and a pinch of salt. Bring it to the boil, then turn the heat down and let it gently simmer for 12–15 minutes, or until all the liquid has been absorbed.

Squeeze out the water from the grated courgette. Put the grated courgette in a bowl with the spring onions, garlic, eggs, lime zest, chives, flour, a large pinch of salt, a grind of pepper and the cooled quinoa. Combine everything with your hands, and put it the fridge for 30 minutes to set. (You can do this the night before you want to eat, ready to cook immediately when you get home the following day.)

Put all the tahini sauce ingredients in a blender, and whizz together.

When you are ready to eat, form the quinoa mix into six patties. Heat 1 tablespoon coconut oil in a frying pan over a high heat, and use a spatula to gently lay the patties in the pan. Cook them for 3–4 minutes on each side.

Serve with the sauce and the cos lettuce leaves used as 'buns'.

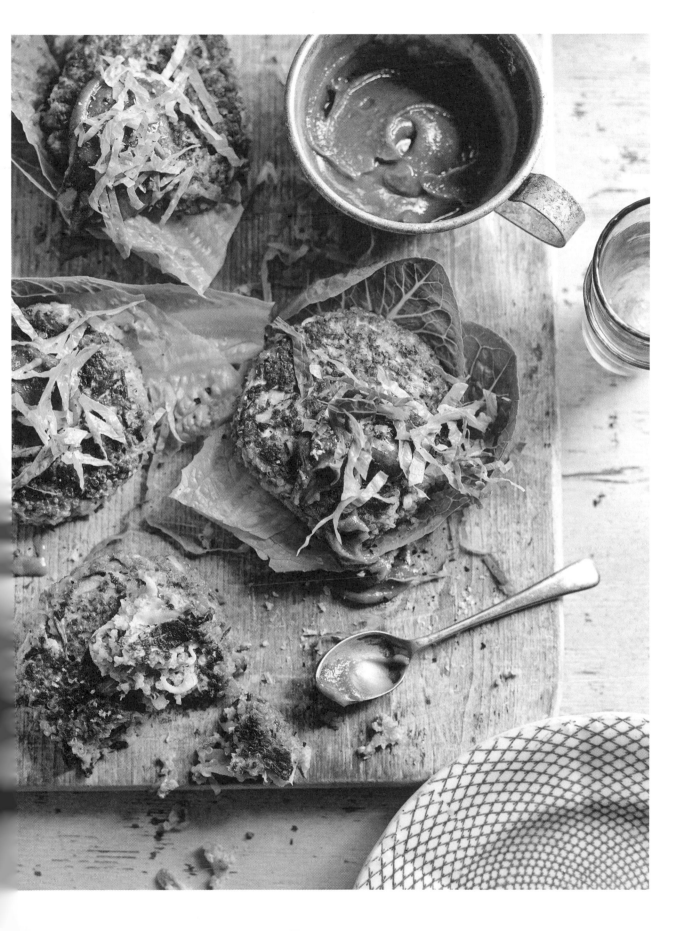

roast lamb shoulder with miso and aubergine, and cauliflower rice

serves 6–8

4 tbsp miso paste
3 tbsp honey
2 tbsp butter or
  coconut oil
2 aubergines, sliced
  lengthways into
  1cm strips
2kg lamb shoulder,
  on the bone
pinch salt
50g sesame seeds
  (optional)

classic plain
cauliflower rice

serves 8

2 cauliflowers,
  stalks removed
  and roughly
  chopped
2 tbsp olive oil
salt and pepper

Slow roast lamb is my speciality; whether you have a slow cooker or not, you can whip this out – no problem! The sweetness of the honey makes the lamb good enough for dessert … you won't see any empty plates with this one.

Put the miso, honey and butter or coconut oil in a saucepan and warm them through for a few minutes.

Set your slow cooker to low, or preheat the oven to 130°C/250°F/ Gas mark ½.

Rub the aubergines in some of the miso mixture, then put them on the bottom of the slow cooker or on the bottom of a large cast-iron pot. Rub the lamb in the rest of the sauce, then put it on top of the aubergines. Throw over a pinch of salt, pop the lid on and cook (whether in the slow cooker or the oven) for 7 hours.

Once done, garnish with sesame seeds, if using, and enjoy this melt-in-the-mouth miso meat. Serve with Classic Plain Cauliflower Rice, below.

classic plain cauliflower rice

Put the roughly chopped cauliflower into a food processor and process for a few minutes until you get a rice-like consistency.

Boil 100ml water in a large saucepan. Throw in the cauliflower rice with a pinch of salt, and cook for 5 minutes, stirring every minute. Drain any excess water and stir in the olive oil and some freshly ground pepper.

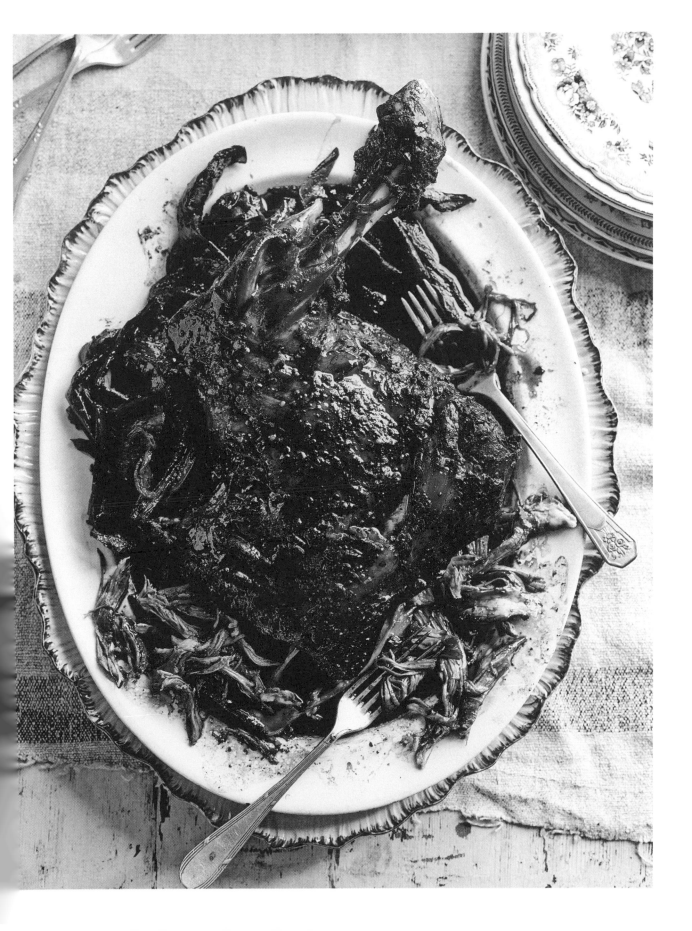

chicken schnitzel with sweet potato fries

serves 2

1 large sweet potato
  or 2 small ones,
  peeled
1 egg, separated
1 tsp smoked
  paprika
4 tbsp coconut oil
50g buckwheat
  flour, rice flour or
  ground almonds
70g buckwheat
  groats
zest and juice of
  1 lemon
1 clove garlic
2 tbsp chopped
  parsley
2 chicken breasts,
  skinned
salt and pepper

You won't see any deep-fried breadcrumbs here ... no, this chicken dish is made with home-ground buckwheat and spiced with garlic and parsley. It goes so well with the sweet potato fries, which are egg-washed to make them nice and crispy without the need for a fryer.

Preheat the oven to 200°C/400°F/Gas mark 6. Slice the sweet potato into chips about 1cm wide. Whisk the egg white for a few seconds. Add salt, pepper and the smoked paprika. Dip the sweet potato chips into the egg white mix, then lay them out on a baking tray. Melt 2 tablespoons coconut oil and pour it over the top of them; toss well so they are covered.

Roast the chips in the oven for 30 minutes, or until cooked through. Give them a stir halfway through so they cook evenly.

Put the flour or ground almonds in a bowl. Whisk the egg yolk with the remainder of the egg white mix in another bowl. Put the buckwheat groats, lemon zest, garlic and parsley in the food processor with a big pinch of salt and some pepper. Blitz for 3–4 minutes, or until broken down into breadcrumb size. Pour this mixture into a bowl and set aside.

Cut the chicken breasts down their length and open them out, and bash with a rolling pin until they are just under 1cm thick. Season the chicken, coat in the flour, then dip them into the egg mix, and finally dip them into the buckwheat crumbs.

Heat 1 tablespoon coconut oil in a frying pan over a medium heat, and cook the chicken for 4 minutes on each side until golden-brown and cooked through. Repeat with the other chicken breast and serve with the sweet potato fries.

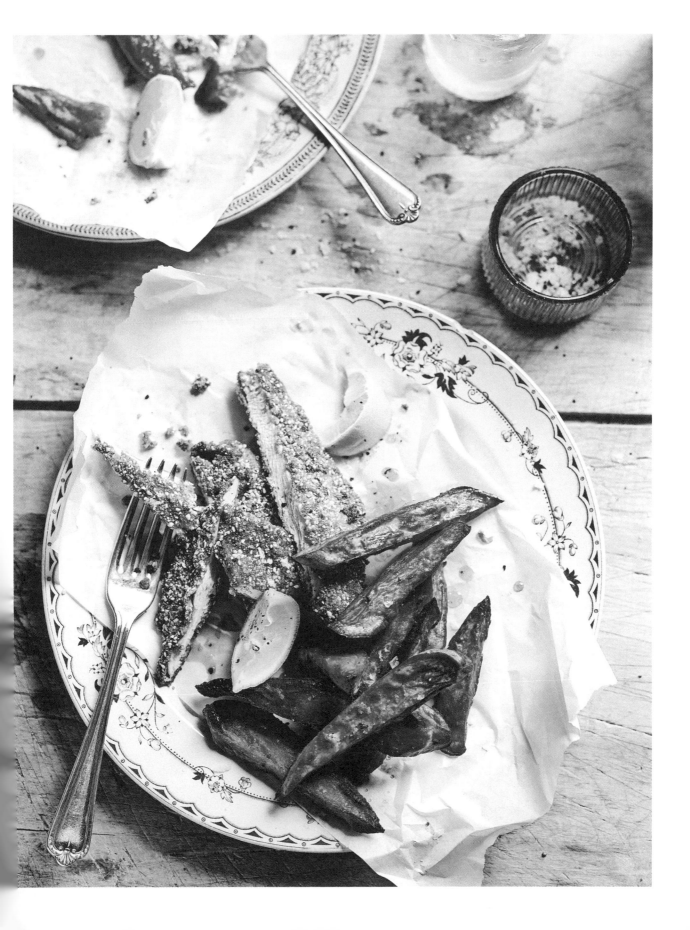

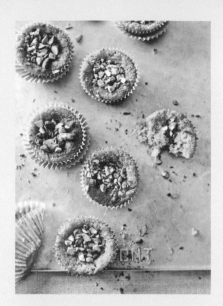

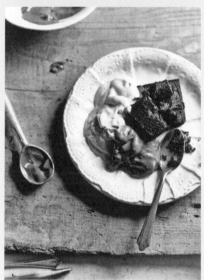

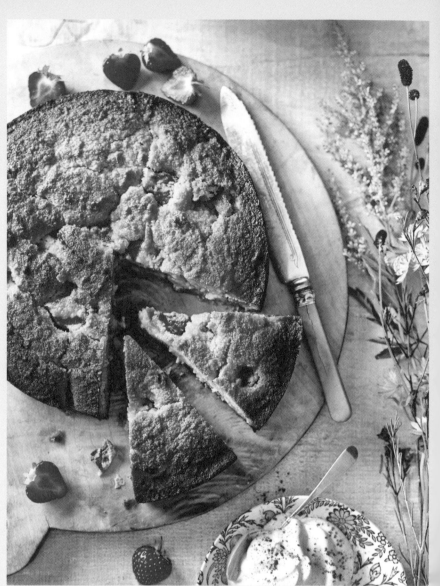

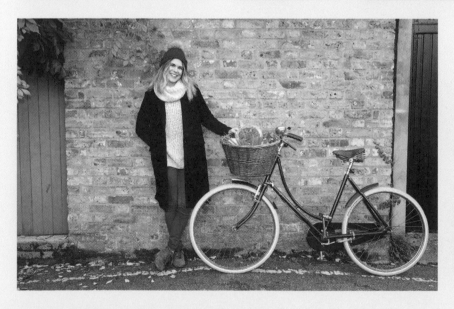

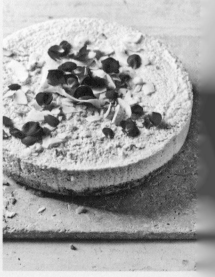

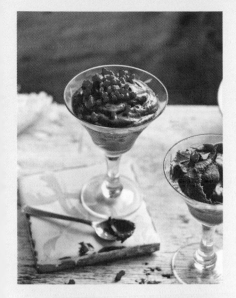

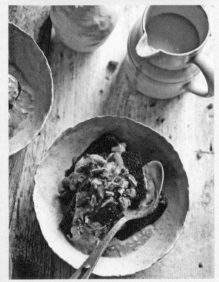

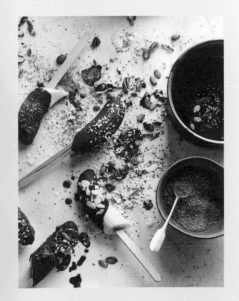

sweet
treats

raw lemon cheesecake

serves 12

400g cashew nuts
200g Medjool
  dates, stoned
200g almond flakes
  or blanched
  almonds
150g desiccated
  coconut
2 tbsp coconut oil
zest of 3 lemons
300ml almond milk
200ml freshly
  squeezed lemon
  juice
160g coconut
  butter
1 tsp vanilla
  powder
260g honey
coconut flakes,
  lightly toasted,
  and rose petals,
  for topping
salt

This recipe calls for coconut butter, sometimes known as coconut manna – it's creamy and oh-so-tasty. This cake is totally raw, and you will find it hard to stop munching your way through it in one sitting.

Soak the cashew nuts in enough water to cover for 4 hours, then drain and set aside.

In a blender, blend the dates, almonds and desiccated coconut with 1 tablespoon coconut oil, a pinch of salt and the zest of 2 lemons. Keep blending until everything is mixed together. Flatten the base into a 25cm cake tin with a removable bottom.

Put the soaked cashew nuts, the almond milk, the lemon juice, the zest of 1 lemon, the coconut butter, a pinch of salt, the vanilla powder, the honey and 1 tablespoon coconut oil into the food processor and whizz until smooth. Pour the mixture on top of the base and put it in the freezer for at least 2 hours, then transfer to the fridge.

Serve with lightly toasted coconut flakes and rose petals.

Note:
All raw desserts in this section will keep for 1–2 weeks in the fridge. All cooked cakes will keep for 2–3 days in the fridge.

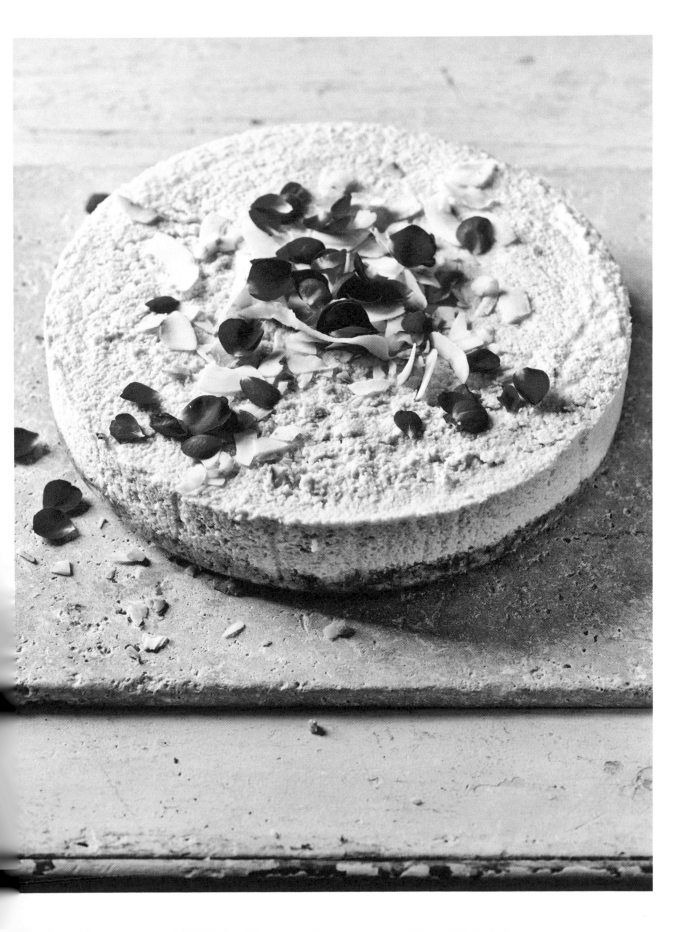

sticky toffee pudding with vanilla custard

serves 4–6

100ml just-boiled
  water
250g dates, stoned
3 eggs
100g coconut oil or
  butter, plus extra
  for greasing
275g ground
  almonds (or other
  gluten-free flour)
1 tbsp bicarbonate
  of soda
pinch sea salt
2 tsp cinnamon
1 tsp ground ginger
2 tbsp honey
4 tbsp pecan nuts,
  crushed
cinnamon, for
  dusting

vanilla custard
500ml almond, rice
  or coconut milk
2 tbsp honey or
  coconut sugar
3 tsp vanilla bean
  paste
6 egg yolks

It's the staple pudding of many a pub or restaurant. But how to make it healthy? This was a challenge I was extremely keen to take on. The result is pure decadence, with dairy-free custard, gooey dates and soft sponge. I think you're going to enjoy making this.

Preheat the oven to 160°C/325°F/Gas mark 3.

Put the just-boiled water and dates in a saucepan over a medium heat, and simmer for 4 minutes. Whizz the dates and liquid in the food processor for 2 minutes, then add the eggs and coconut oil or butter and blitz again. Gently fold in the ground almonds, bicarbonate of soda, salt and spices until fully combined.

Grease a 900g loaf tin with coconut oil or butter, and spoon the mixture in. Place a bit of foil over the top of the dish. Pop it in the oven for 35 minutes. For the last 5–10 minutes take the foil off so the top gets a good roasting.

For the custard, heat the milk, honey or coconut sugar, and vanilla in a small saucepan over a medium to high heat. Beat the egg yolks in a bowl, then pour the milk (just before it boils) over the top and whisk well. When everything is combined, pour it back into the pan over a low heat. Keep whisking until the custard thickens a little. Remove it from the heat and put it back into the bowl to cool.

Take the pudding out of the oven and put it on a cooling rack. (Leave it in the tin.) Melt the honey over a low heat and pour this evenly over the top (spread it with a knife), then sprinkle on the pecan nuts. Enjoy with a dollop of custard and a dusting of cinnamon.

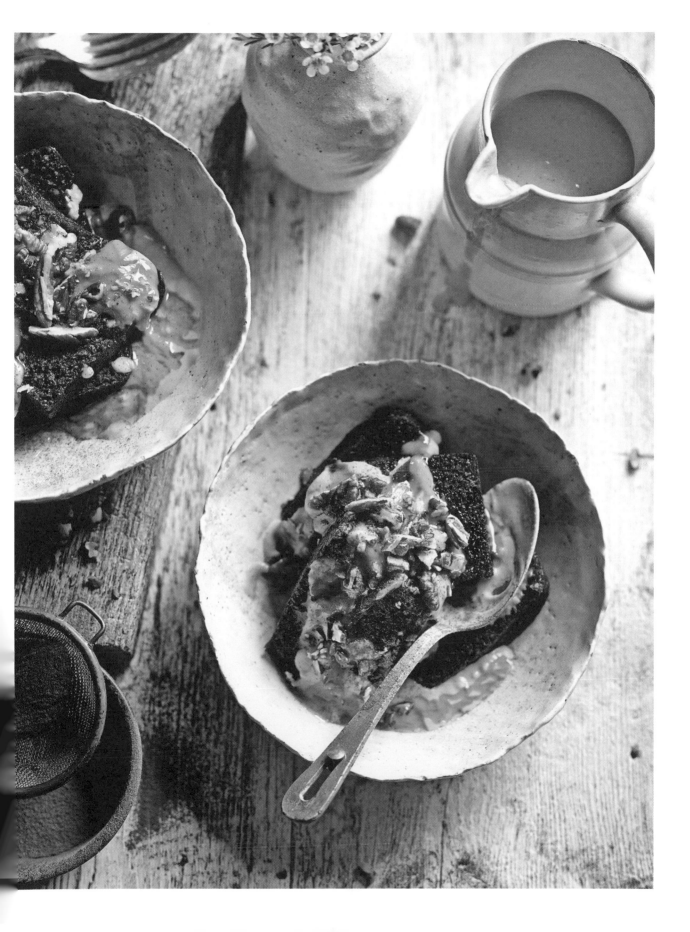

red velvet cupcakes with coconut whipped cream

makes 18 cupcakes

250g buckwheat
    flour (or other
    gluten-free flour)
3 tbsp raw cacao
    powder
1 tsp cinnamon,
    plus extra for
    dusting
2 tsp baking
    powder
½ tsp bicarbonate
    of soda
200g butter
250g coconut sugar
    or honey
2 small beetroots,
    finely grated
1 tsp vanilla extract
2 large eggs
150ml coconut milk
    (or other milk of
    your choice)

This is essentially the dream cupcake without the usual associated guilt. Beetroot acts as the food dye, so there's no need to worry about preservatives. Then there is the gluten-free buckwheat flour acting as the base. The outcome is quite lovely.

Preheat the oven to 160°C/325°F/Gas mark 3.

Line two cupcake tins with 18 paper cases. In a bowl combine the flour, cacao, cinnamon, baking powder and bicarbonate of soda. Use the food processor to cream the butter and coconut sugar or honey for a few minutes, until light and fluffy, then add the beetroot and vanilla. Pour the contents of the food processor into the dry ingredients. Add the eggs one by one, and finally the milk, stirring vigorously.

Bake for 18 minutes, then let the cupcakes cool before topping them with Coconut Whipped Cream (see page 222) and finishing with a dusting of cinnamon.

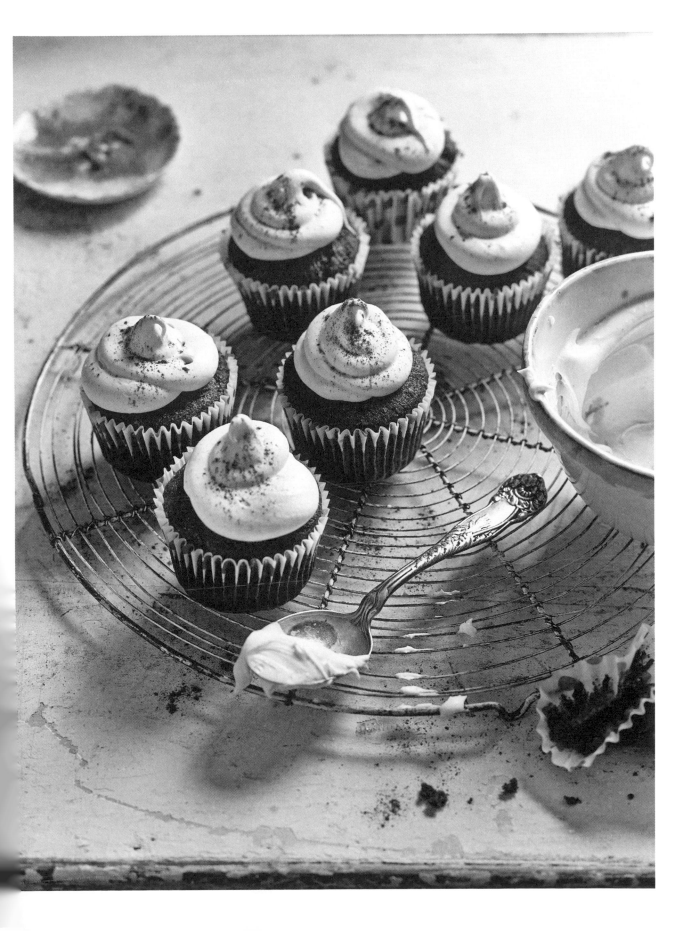

coconut whipped cream

This cream is fun, light and a great dairy-free alternative, full of healthy fats. It also has fertility boosting properties, and helps to replenish the skin, keeping it youthful and glowing.

serves 12–18 (as an accompaniment)

1 x 400ml can coconut milk
½ tsp cinnamon

To make the coconut cream, place the unopened, upside-down can of coconut milk in the fridge, and leave it overnight. (You may want to do this the day before you want to serve the cream.) Place a bowl in the fridge next to it.

Open the can and drain out the coconut milk that has separated from the cream. Place the milk in a glass (this can be used to make smoothies, or drunk while you make the whipped cream.

Scoop the cream out of the can and put it into the chilled bowl, then whip it with a handheld electric mixer until it fluffs up. Add the cinnamon, and whip again.

You can also add honey, raw cacao or vanilla to the whipped coconut cream for more flavour and sweetness.

dairy-free neapolitan ice cream

This dish reminds me of my childhood – after dinner at Pizza Express we would always tuck into some Neapolitan to finish the night off. This ice cream (pictured overleaf) is super-simple; it doesn't require a fancy ice-cream maker and is as nutritious as it is delicious.

serves 2
1 x 400ml can coconut milk
3 bananas, peeled and frozen overnight
1 tbsp raw cacao powder
5 frozen strawberries
1 vanilla pod

Open the can of coconut milk, and mix the cream and milk together if they have separated.

To make the chocolate ice cream: Mix one of the bananas with one-third of the coconut milk and the cacao powder in the food processor until you have an ice-cream consistency, and pop it into a bowl.

To make the vanilla ice cream: Mix one of the bananas with one-third of the coconut milk and the whole vanilla pod in the food processor until you have an ice-cream consistency, and pop it into a bowl.

To make the strawberry ice cream: Mix one of the bananas with one-third of the coconut milk and the strawberries in the food processor until you have an ice-cream consistency, and pop it into a bowl.

Plate all three ice creams together.

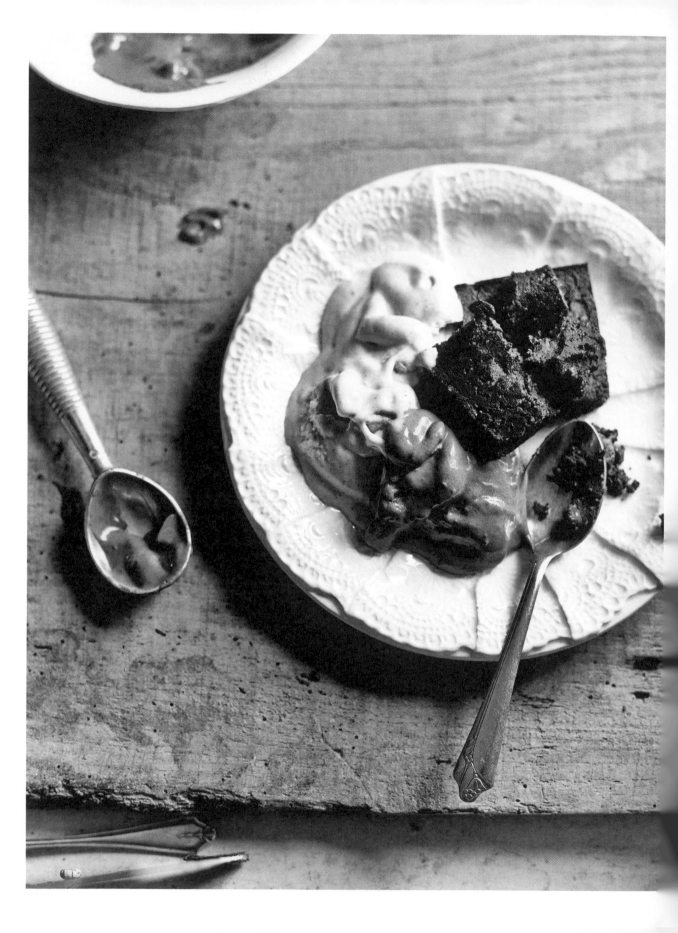

raw chocolate brownies

This is my favourite guilt-free treat. The hazelnuts give this a rich, indulgent feel, which, combined with the energy-boosting raw cacao powder, will keep you coming back for more after just one bite.

serves 6

150g hazelnuts
150g Medjool dates, stoned
small pinch salt
50g raw cacao powder
3 tbsp coconut oil

In a blender or food processor, blend the hazelnuts for 3 minutes then add the dates, salt and cacao. Slowly add the coconut oil as the mixture is blending. Allow this to mix in for a few minutes. Once the mixture is totally blended together, use a spatula to scrape the mixture into a square cake tin or baking dish. Put the mixture in the freezer for 30 minutes, then refrigerate until you want to serve it. It goes perfectly with my Dairy-Free Neapolitan Ice Cream (see recipe page 223).

raw cherry and chocolate fudge

If you struggle to fall asleep, cherry can be a great sleep aid – and the raw gooey texture makes this fudge a perfect treat with a cup of chamomile tea before bed. Don't forget the active ingredient, almond butter – it provides lots of vitamin E for your skin.

serves 6
100g almond butter (or any other nut butter)
100g coconut oil, plus extra for greasing
50g raw cacao powder
100g honey
1 tsp vanilla extract
pinch sea salt
50g dried cherries

Put the nut butter and coconut oil in the food processor and mix for 1 minute or so. Sieve in the raw cacao, then put in the rest of the ingredients (apart from the cherries) and whizz for a few minutes until totally gooey. At this point throw in the cherries and mix with a spoon.

Scoop out the mixture with a spatula into a coconut oil-greased 24cm baking tin, then put it in the freezer for 30 minutes until firmly set.

Cut the fudge into bite-size pieces with a sharp knife, then pop them back in the fridge.

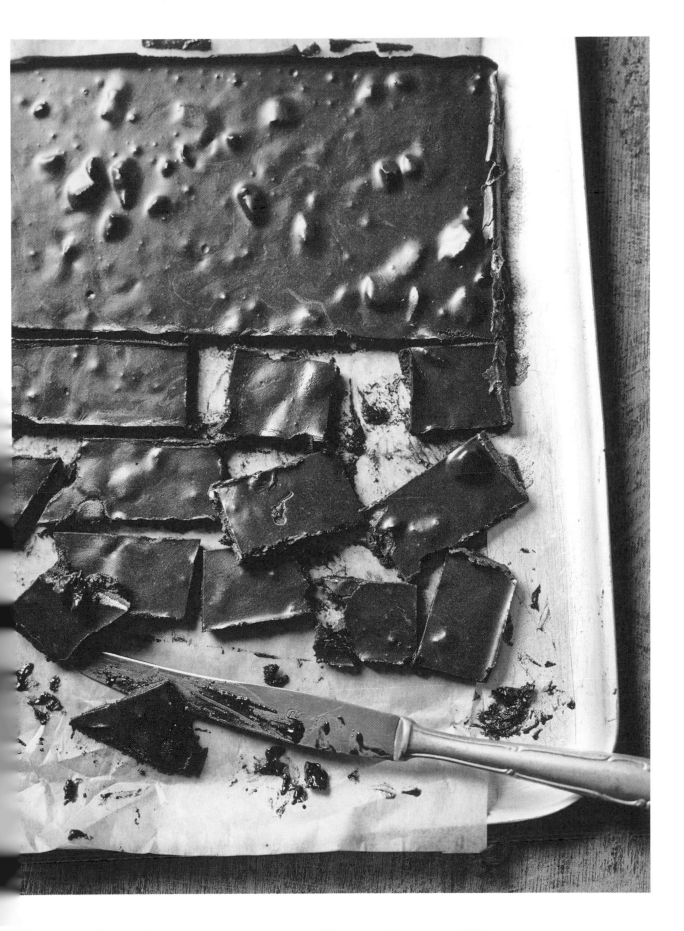

banana and cinnamon loaf

This is a healthy spin on my boyfriend's banana bread recipe, which is famous at his restaurant in London. I swapped a few things around to make it glowified, and it works a treat. You can have this for breakfast, too. In Sydney I used to have banana bread with coconut flesh for breakfast all the time.

serves 6–8

1 vanilla pod
110g butter or coconut oil, melted
250g coconut sugar
4 ripe bananas
4 tbsp almond milk, rice milk, coconut milk or whole milk
1 egg
1 tsp baking powder
½ tsp bicarbonate of soda
275g rice flour, ground almonds or buckwheat flour
1 tsp cinnamon

Preheat the oven to 180°C/350°F/Gas mark 4.

Cut open the vanilla pod and scrape out the seeds. Mix all the ingredients together in the food processor. Pour into a 900g loaf tin lined with baking paper, and bake for 50 minutes, until almost cooked through.

Remove the loaf from the tin and leave it to cool, then dig in.

Serve with a smear of my homemade Chocolate Hazelnut Spread (see page 86) or Chia Raspberry Jam (see page 85).

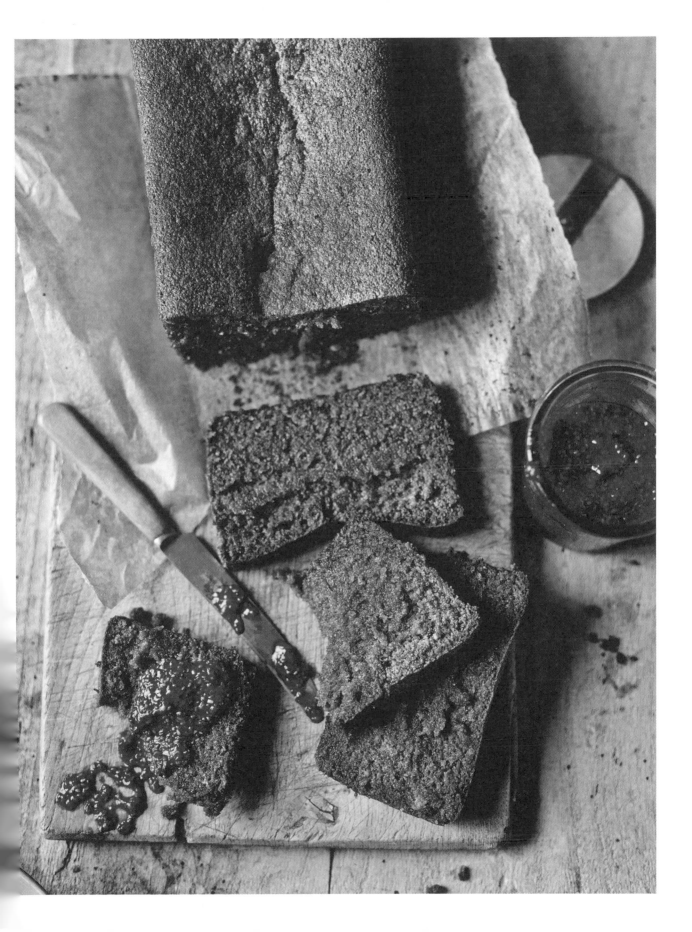

raw chocolate avocado mousse

Do it by numbers! This is the perfect dinner party dessert, as you can make it for plenty with satisfaction guaranteed. Some people worry about avocado being in a dessert, but trust me on this one – it creates a rich velvety texture unrivalled by any unhealthy alternatives.

serves 2

1 ripe avocado, stoned and flesh scooped out
1 ripe banana, peeled
3 tbsp coconut oil
4 tbsp raw cacao powder
pinch sea salt
100ml almond milk, coconut milk or rice milk, plus extra if needed
1 handful frozen raspberries

Put the avocado, banana, coconut oil, cacao powder and salt in the blender, and blend. Slowly add the milk until the mixture becomes creamy and easily moves around the blender; add a little extra milk if the mixture isn't creamy enough.

Pour the mousse into two ramekins or cocktail glasses, then put them in the freezer for 30 minutes before transferring to the fridge.

Crumble the raspberries in your hands over the top of each dessert, and enjoy. Top with a little honey for some added sweetness.

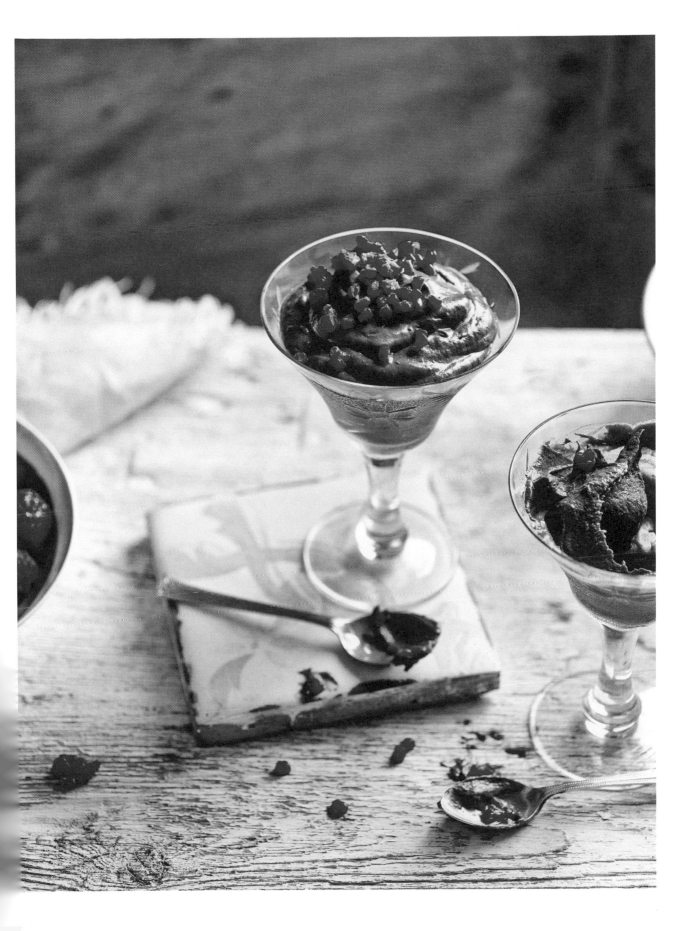

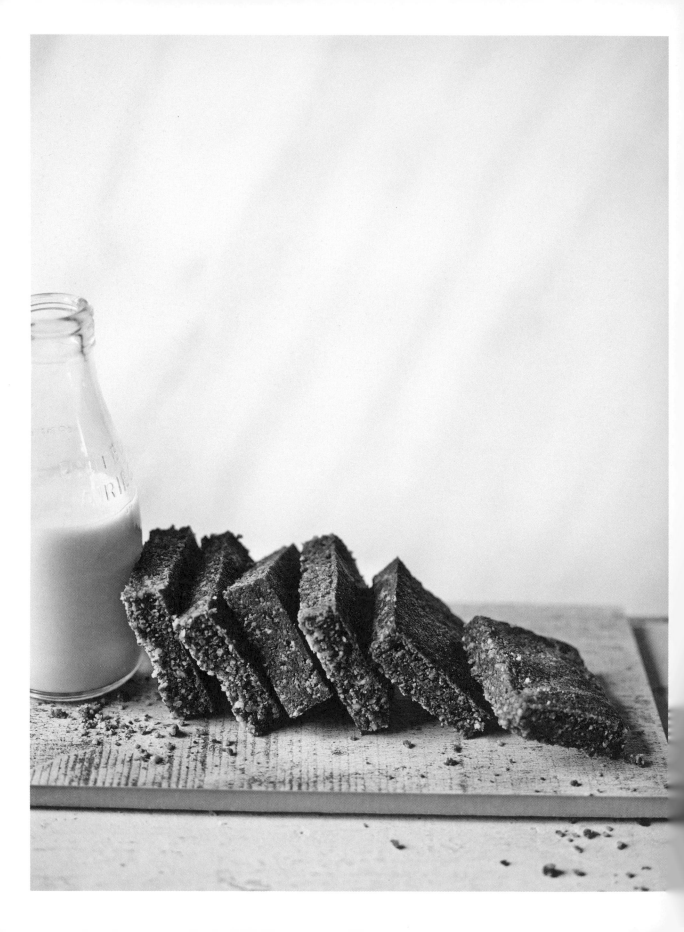

the super-healthy flapjack

This is a perfect pre-workout snack, or to sustain you at the 4pm slump. It's totally grain free, and is packed full of protein-rich nuts.

makes 16 squares

200g pecan nuts
300g hazelnuts
150g dates, stoned
1 ripe banana, peeled
4 tbsp honey
150g sunflower seeds
30g coconut oil or butter
1½ tbsp cinnamon
1½ tbsp ground ginger
coconut oil or butter, for greasing
pinch sea salt

Preheat the oven to 180°C/350°F/Gas mark 4.

In a food processor, blitz the nuts for 30 seconds to 1 minute – until lightly ground. Put the ground nuts in a bowl. Put the rest of the flapjack ingredients into the food processor and whizz for a few minutes, then pour this over the nuts and stir with a wooden spoon until fully combined.

Put the mixture into a small (approximately 24 x 35cm) baking tray greased with coconut oil or butter and lined with baking paper, and bake for 20–25 minutes. (You're aiming for crispy on the outside and gooey on the inside!)

Take the flapjacks out of the oven, remove them from the tin and let them cool before you cut into them.

date and pistachio cookies

These are my Middle Eastern-inspired cookies.
I use coconut sugar to sweeten them; this delectable
treat comes from the sap of the coconut, and is a very
sustainable sweetener. I can't tell you how much
I love these!

serves 6

200g coconut sugar
125g butter or coconut oil
1 egg, beaten
250g buckwheat flour (or other gluten-free flour)
½ tsp salt
½ tsp baking powder
50g raw unsalted pistachios, roughly chopped
50g dates, stoned and chopped

Preheat the oven to 160°C/325°F/Gas mark 3.

In a food processor cream the coconut sugar and butter or coconut
oil, then put the mixture in a bowl. Add the beaten egg to the
creamed butter and sugar, mixing gently. Slowly add the flour,
a little at a time, and fold in with a spoon.

Finally, add the salt, baking powder, pistachios and dates, and mix
everything together well.

Roll the dough into 12 walnut-size balls, and put them onto a baking
tray lined with baking paper. Slightly flatten each ball into a cookie
shape.

Bake for 8 minutes, then let them cool for 10 minutes . . . and enjoy.

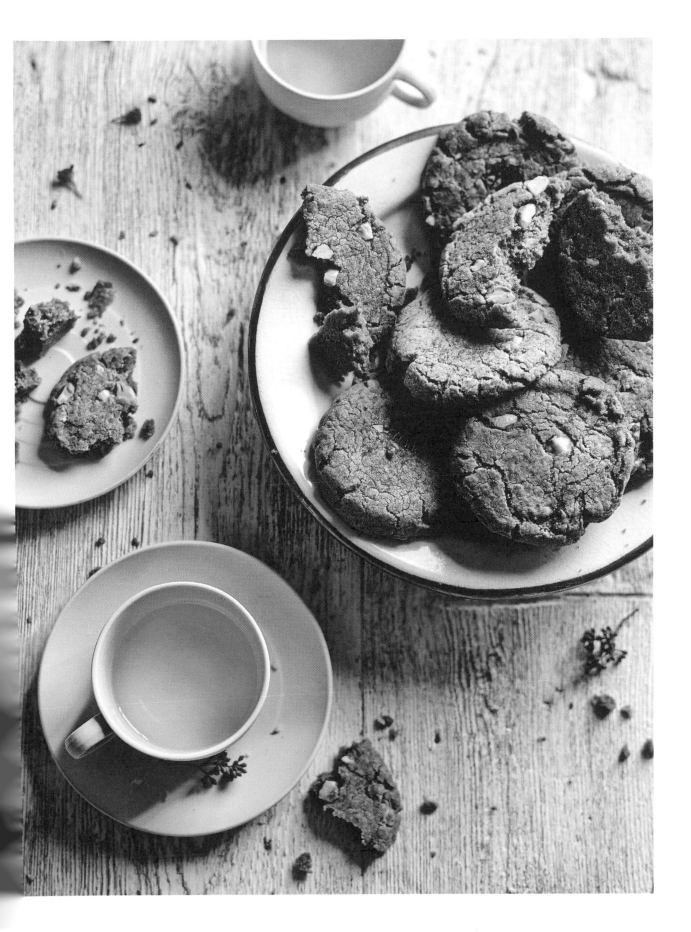

ginger cookie cups

Cookies and milk … so reminiscent of my childhood. This recipe merges them together, by creating a cookie cup that gets filled with milk. It looks awesome and is a fun spin on your typical cookie. Spiced with ginger, these cookies have a nice earthy feel from the oats and sweetness from the coconut sugar.

serves 6

200g coconut sugar
150g butter or coconut oil, plus extra for greasing
1 egg
275g oats
½ tsp salt
1 tbsp ground ginger
250ml almond milk and berries of your choice, to serve

Preheat the oven to 180°C/350°F/Gas mark 4.

In a food processor cream the coconut sugar and butter or coconut oil, then put the mixture in a bowl. Add the egg to the creamed butter and sugar, processing gently. Throw in the oats, salt and ginger, and pulse for a few minutes more until the mixture forms a dough.

Grab a couple of cupcake tins, grease them with butter or coconut oil and divide the dough evenly into 16. Press the dough to the bottom of the moulds, allowing for it to move up the sides to form a cup-like shape. Keep the cookie layer around ½cm thick.

Bake for 10–12 minutes, then let the cups cool.

Pour in the almond milk, then scatter with berries and enjoy.

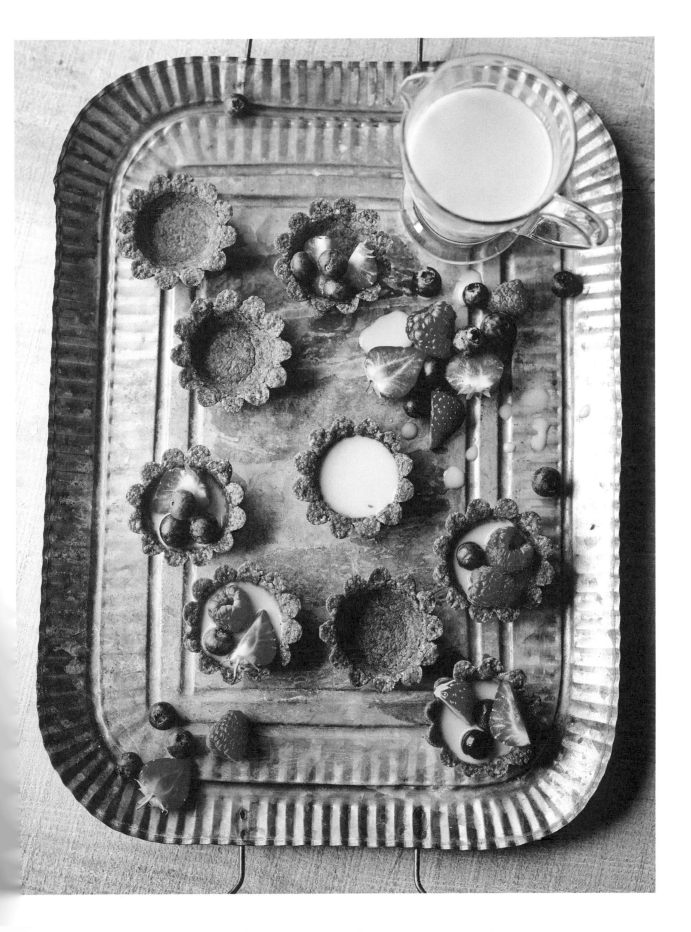

cherry crumble with cashew nut cream

serves 6

600g cherries (or
  other berries),
  stalks removed
  and stoned
1 tbsp honey
1 tsp cinnamon
1 tsp grated
  nutmeg
zest and juice of
  1 orange
100g almonds
200g oats
small pinch sea salt
75g coconut oil or
  butter
100g walnuts

cashew nut cream
150g cashew nuts
150ml water or
  coconut water
½ tsp vanilla
  extract or powder
½ tsp cinnamon
tiny pinch salt
1 Medjool date,
  stoned (optional)

Cherries remind me of long summer nights, and this nutty crumble takes them to another level. I have added some extra nutty goodness to the crumble to up your vitamin E intake and make sure that glow is happening all night long.

Preheat the oven to 180°C/350°F/Gas mark 4.

Put the cherries, honey, cinnamon, nutmeg and orange zest and juice in a saucepan. Heat over a medium heat for 5–8 minutes, or until the cherries soften.

Put the almonds, oats, pinch of salt, coconut oil or butter, and walnuts in a food processor and grind them for 30 seconds until they are slightly ground but still crunchy.

Place the cherry mixture into a 900g loaf tin with tall sides, then scatter the nut crumble on top. Bake for 25–30 minutes, until the top is slightly golden.

To make the cashew nut cream, put all the ingredients in a blender, and blend for 3–5 minutes until totally creamy. Serve together while the crumble is still hot.

When cherries aren't available, switch to 200g cooking apples and 200g mixed berries.

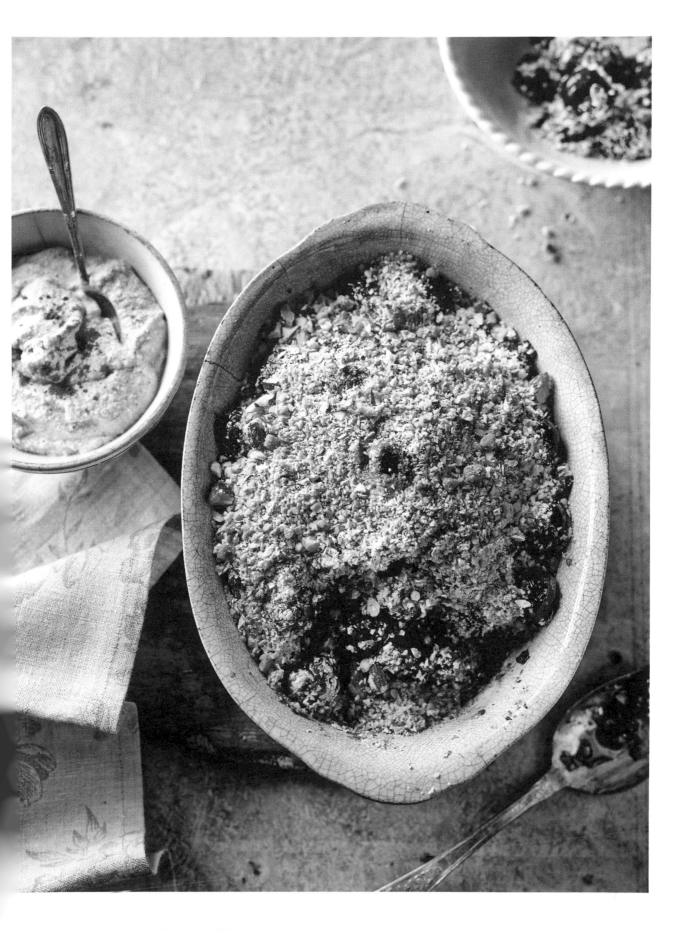

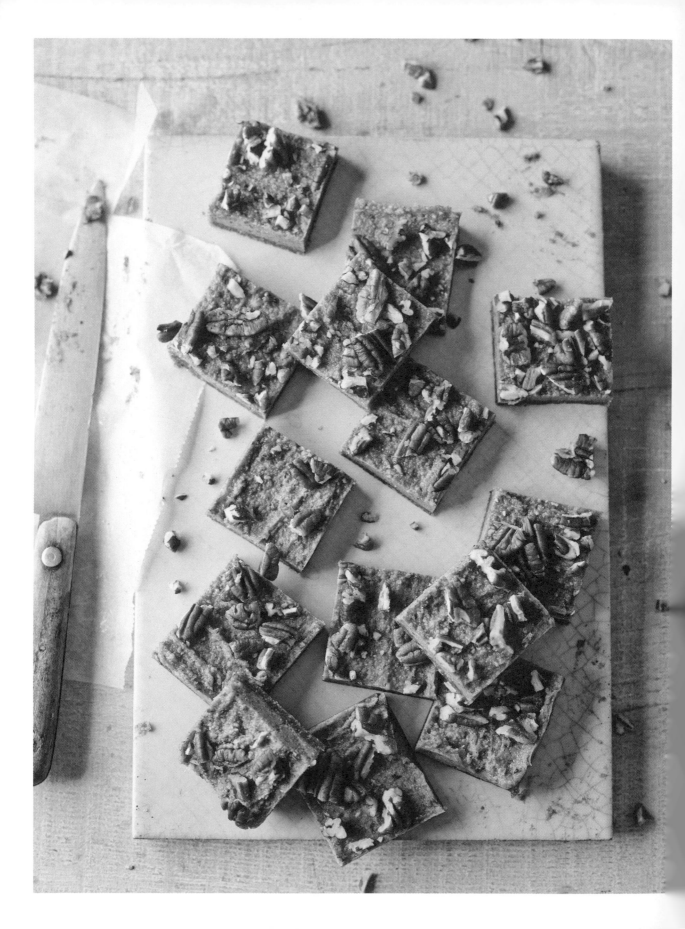

pecan pie bites

I always find that mini bites are great for bigger groups and marvellous for sharing. Texture from the pecan nuts gives the soft base a wonderful balance, with the perfect blend of date and cinnamon.

Chop up 150g dates into small pieces. Soak the chopped dates in the just-boiled water and set aside.

To make the crust, put 100g pecan nuts in the food processor with the almonds, desiccated coconut, 1 tablespoon coconut oil, salt and 150g non-soaked dates. Whizz for a few minutes. Grease a small baking tray or cake tin (approximately 23 x 35cm) with coconut oil and pour the crust mix into it; spread it over the bottom to create a 2.5cm-thick crust.

Once cooled, pour the soaked dates into the blender along with with the soaking water, 200g pecan nuts, 4 tablespoons coconut oil, cinnamon, milk and honey. Blend for a few minutes until smooth, then pour over the crust.

Arrange the rest of the pecan nuts on top and pop the whole thing in the freezer for 1 hour to harden. Cut into bite-size pieces and transfer to the fridge.

This will keep in the fridge for 10 days.

serves 8

300g Medjool dates, stoned
50ml just-boiled water
350g pecan nuts
50g almonds
50g desiccated coconut
5 tbsp coconut oil, plus extra for greasing
pinch salt
1 tsp cinnamon
50ml almond milk, rice milk or oat milk
2 tbsp honey

pear and almond tart

serves 8

pears
300ml water
1 vanilla pod
1 tbsp ground
  cinnamon
100g honey
4 pears, peeled,
  cored and cut in
  half

crust
small pinch salt
50g butter or
  coconut oil, plus
  extra for greasing
1 tbsp honey
1 tsp vanilla extract
  or powder
1 egg
200g ground
  almonds

filling
120g ground
  almonds
150g honey
3 eggs
125g butter or
  coconut oil

toasted almonds
  and fresh berries,
  to serve

I love pastry. In fact I am a pastry fiend. This almond crispy crust goes perfectly with the soft, melt-in-your-mouth pears. Make this one for a nice afternoon treat on the weekend.

Preheat the oven to 160°C/325°F/Gas mark 3.

Put the water, vanilla, cinnamon and honey in a small saucepan and bring to a high simmer, then add the pears and let them poach with the lid on for 20 minutes.

Meanwhile, make the crust. Blitz all the crust ingredients apart from the ground almonds in the food processor, then slowly fold in the ground almonds. Grease a 26cm pie dish with some butter or coconut oil, and tip the crust into it. Spread the mix out evenly and use your hands to press it up the side of the tin. With a fork, prick the pastry base. Cook for 10–15 minutes, until bronzed.

Meanwhile, make the filling. Blend the ground almonds, honey, eggs, and butter or coconut oil.

When the base is ready, pour in the filling. Place the poached pears on top, then bake for 30 minutes.

Serve topped with toasted almonds and fresh berries.

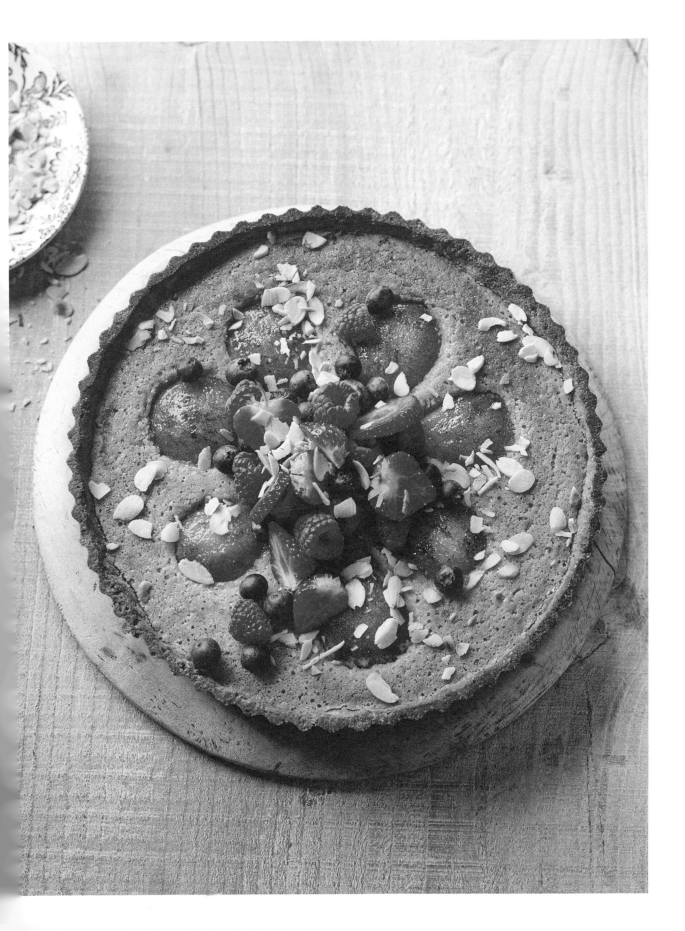

strawberry cake with coconut whipped cream

serves 12

170g butter or
  coconut oil, plus
  extra for greasing
300g ground
  almonds (or
  gluten-free flour)
1 tsp baking
  powder
170g coconut sugar
  or honey
1 tsp vanilla extract
3 large eggs
300g strawberries,
  hulled and cut in
  half

This is my take on a classic almond cake, with the freshness of ripe berries. It sits well with the coconut cream, creating a lingering finish. You'll need to start the Coconut Whipped Cream (see page 222) the day before you make the cake.

Preheat the oven to 160°C/325°F/Gas mark 3. Generously grease a 23cm cake tin with butter or coconut oil and line with baking paper.

Mix the ground almonds or gluten-free flour and baking powder in a large bowl. Put the butter or coconut oil, coconut sugar or honey and vanilla into the food processor, and blitz until light and fluffy. Add the eggs, one at a time, mixing to incorporate, then slowly add the flour. Transfer the cake mix to a bowl, and fold in the strawberries. Stir well together, pour into the cake tin and bake for 45 minutes.

Serve with the Coconut Whipped Cream (page 222).

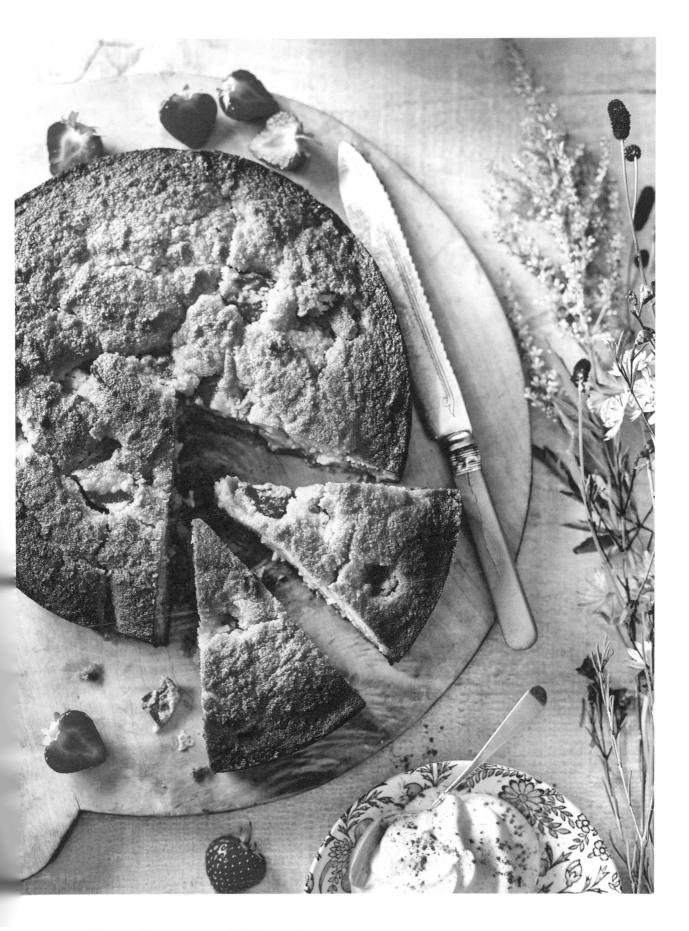

lemon cupcakes with pistachios

Cupcakes always bring joy to my life. The freshness and zing of lemon with that subtle crunch of pistachio make these cupcakes a perfect treat or afternoon snack.

makes 8

170g ground almonds
1 tsp bicarbonate of soda
pinch salt
zest of 3 lemons, juice of 2 lemons
70g honey or coconut sugar
70g butter or coconut oil
3 large free-range eggs
50g raw pistachios, finely chopped,
  plus extra for topping

Preheat the oven to 180°C/350°F/Gas mark 4. Grease 8 paper cupcake holders.

Mix the ground almonds, bicarbonate of soda, salt and lemon zest in a bowl. In a food processor, mix the honey or coconut sugar with the butter or coconut oil, then slowly add the eggs one at a time, then the lemon juice. Pour this on top of the ground almond mixture, and mix together well. Pour the cake batter into the cupcake holders, then sprinkle the pistachios over the top.

Bake for 18–20 minutes. When out of the oven, sprinkle more pistachios on top.

These cupcakes will keep for a few days in an airtight container.

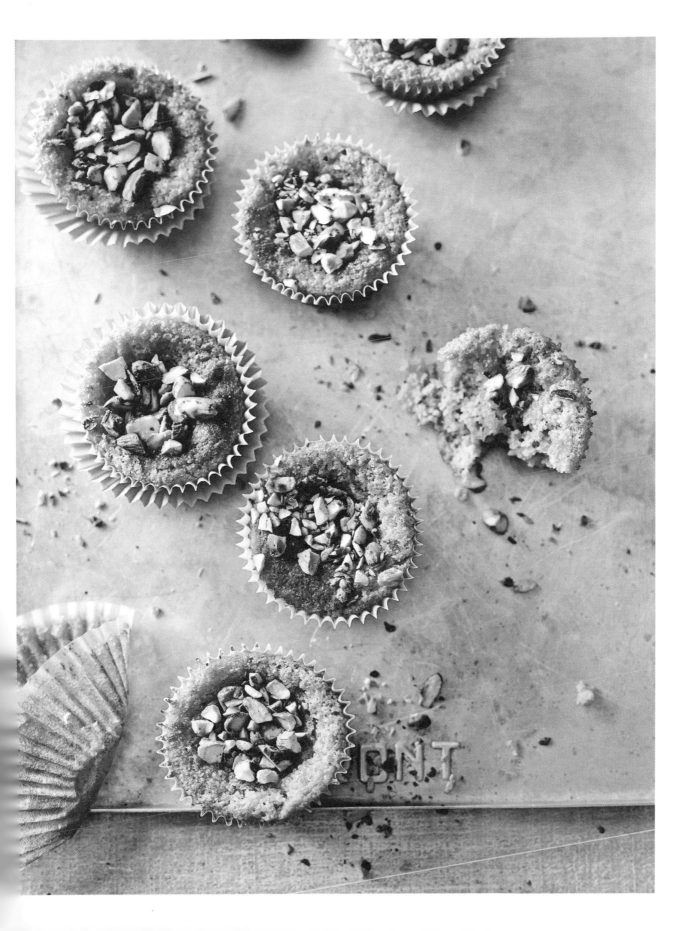

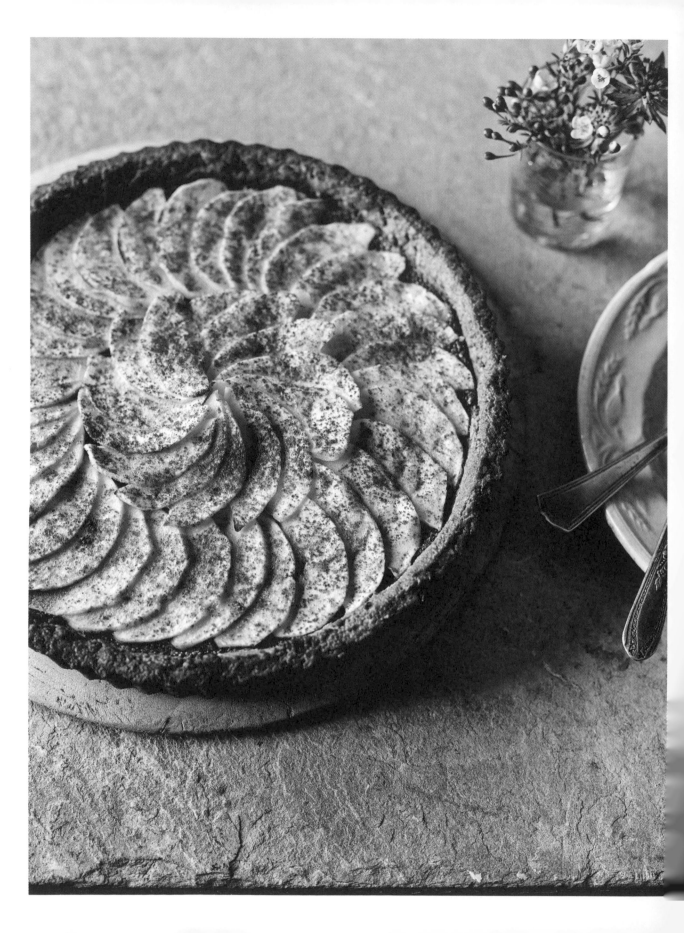

apple tart

While this dessert is already a classic, my version showcases numerous superfoods that extend its possibilities! Chia seeds act as a binding agent, marrying the apple and sugar-level-regulating cinnamon to create the perfect guilt-free pie.

Preheat the oven to 150°C/300°F/Gas mark 2.

To make the base, blitz the walnuts in a food processor until there are no big chunks left. Add the rest of the ingredients for the base and blend until you have a dough-like texture. Roll out the pastry on a lightly floured surface. Trim the dough to fit the top of your tin and leave a slight overhang.

Grease a 26cm round loose-base baking tin. Use your rolling pin to transfer the pastry to the tin, then push it into the tin. Set aside while you make the filling.

Blend the pears with the chia seeds, lemon zest and honey. Leave this for 15 minutes to form a gel.

Cut the apples into quarters, and slice them very thinly. Cover the crust with half of the apple. Dust half of the cinnamon and dot the butter or coconut oil over the top.

Spoon the pear and chia gel on top of the apple layer, and then arrange the rest of the sliced apples on top. Sprinkle over the rest of the cinnamon and butter or coconut oil, and bake in the oven for 25–30 minutes until the top is bronzed.

Once cooked to your desired crispness, remove from the oven and allow to cool. Dust with cinnamon to serve.

serves 8

base
200g walnuts
75g desiccated coconut
80g dates, stoned (I prefer Medjool)
3 tbsp butter or coconut oil, plus extra for greasing
1 tbsp honey
1 tbsp cinnamon
pinch salt
1 tsp crushed vanilla pod or 1 drop extract
2 eggs
zest of 1 lemon
gluten-free flour, for dusting

filling
3 pears, peeled and cored
100g chia seeds
zest of 1 lemon
3 tbsp honey
2 large green cooking apples, peeled and cored
1 tbsp cinnamon
1 tbsp butter or coconut oil
cinnamon, to serve

chocolate-dipped bananas

This is the perfect dessert to make in good company, if you want some fun – perhaps with younger relatives. It's so simple and easy. Don't just stick with bananas – try different kinds of fruit. You'll have a great time!

makes 4
2 bananas, peeled and halved across
100g cacao butter (chopped into small chunks)
30g raw cacao powder
2 tbsp honey or coconut sugar
1 tsp vanilla extract or vanilla powder
tiny pinch salt
desiccated coconut, nuts, seeds, to serve

Stick lolly sticks gently into the bottom of the banana where you cut across. Put them in the freezer overnight, or for at least 3–4 hours.

In a saucepan, melt the cacao butter over a very low heat, stirring constantly. Pour in the rest of the ingredients, except for the coconut and the seeds, and keep stirring.

Grab your banana sticks from the freezer. Tilt the pan to the side and dip the bananas in. You have to be quick to decorate them, as the chocolate freezes quickly, so throw some desiccated coconut, nuts, seeds – whatever you like – on top and then set aside. You can always double-dunk if you are too slow the first time!

Repeat for the other bananas.

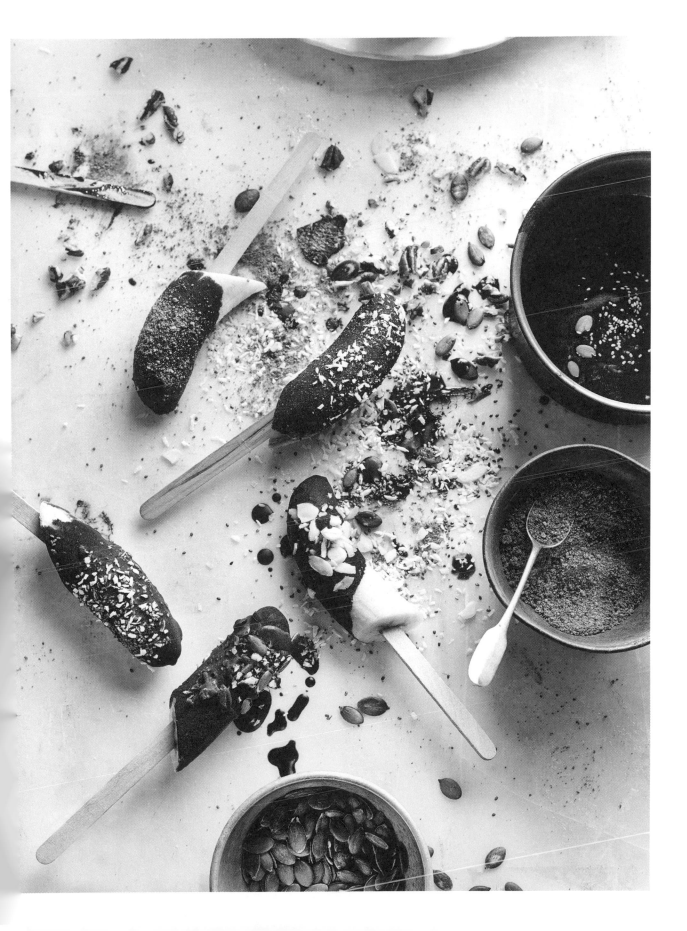

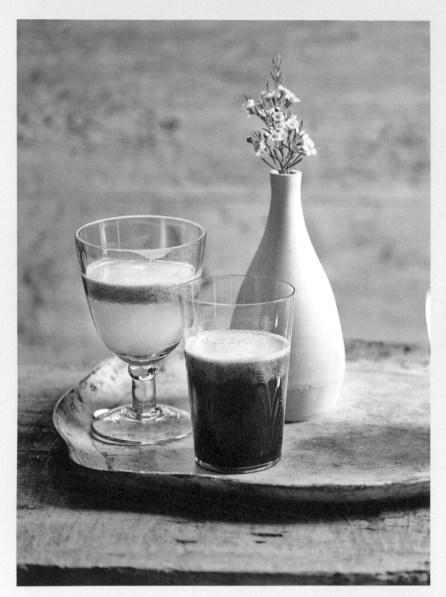
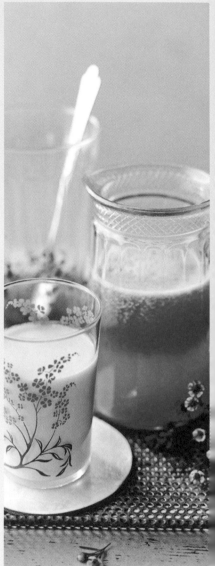
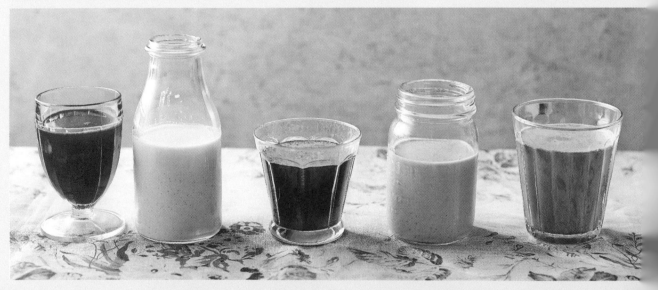

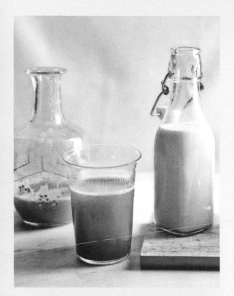

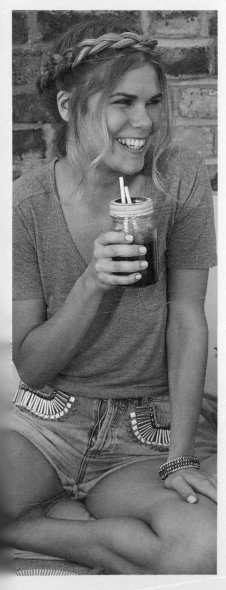

drinks
to
glow

energise

These three juices are packed full of vitamins that will get you bounding out the front door and into the gym. All serve one person.

pre-workout

4 medium carrots
2 beetroots
2 handfuls parsley

2cm piece ginger, peeled

Put all the ingredients into a juicer. Drink that day.

eternal energy

1 lemon, peeled and pith
 removed
3 Granny Smith apples,
 peeled and cored
2.5cm piece ginger, peeled
1 cucumber
1 tsp spirulina

Put all the ingredients into a juicer. Drink that day.

4pm pick-me-up

1 handful spinach
5 romaine lettuce leaves
½ cucumber
4 sticks celery
1 lemon, peeled and pith
 removed
1 apple, peeled and cored
2cm piece ginger, peeled
½ tsp cinnamon

Put all the ingredients into a juicer. Drink that day.

cashew milk

This milk can be enjoyed as a dessert or after dinner, for that little sweet kick you know you need.

100g cashew nuts
1 vanilla pod
300ml water
1 tsp honey
tiny pinch salt

Soak the cashew nuts in enough water to cover for 4 hours.

Discard the cashew soaking water, and rinse the cashews in a sieve under running water.

Cut the vanilla pod in half lengthways and scrape out the seeds. Put the soaked cashew nuts, 300ml water, vanilla seeds, honey and salt in a blender. Blend for 3–4 minutes.

The milk will keep for a week in a container in the fridge.

strong and lean smoothie

This is the perfect pre- or post-gym muscle booster. Packed with natural protein from peanut butter and raw protein powder, it's quick and easy to make and will keep hunger at bay for hours.

1 frozen banana (peeled and frozen the night before)
250ml nut milk, rice milk, coconut milk or coconut water
1 tbsp raw protein powder
1 tbsp peanut butter or other nut butter
1 tsp vanilla powder or extract

Blend and enjoy. This is best drunk fresh.

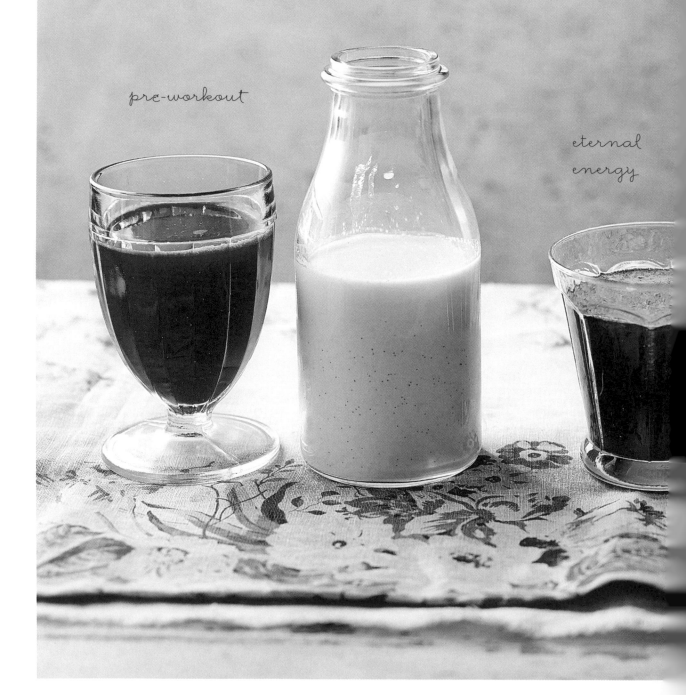

pre-workout

cashew milk

eternal
energy

strong & lean
smoothie

4pm pick-me-up

cleanse

Cleanse your gorgeous body with these nutrient-packed drinks. They're all designed to flush out toxins and reboot your day. All serve one person.

classic cleanse

1 handful parsley
3 medium carrots
1 small beetroot with
  leaves
200g rocket
2 sticks celery

Put all the ingredients into a juicer. Drink that day.

fat buster

¼ watermelon, skin and
  seeds removed
  2 limes, peeled and pith
  removed

Put both ingredients into a juicer. Drink that day.

coconut milk

100g desiccated coconut
150ml water, boiled and
  cooled in the fridge
150ml cold water
pinch salt

Put all the ingredients in a blender. Blend for 4 minutes, then strain through a nut milk bag or piece of muslin. Squeeze the cloth to extract excess liquid.

The milk will keep for a week in a container in the fridge.

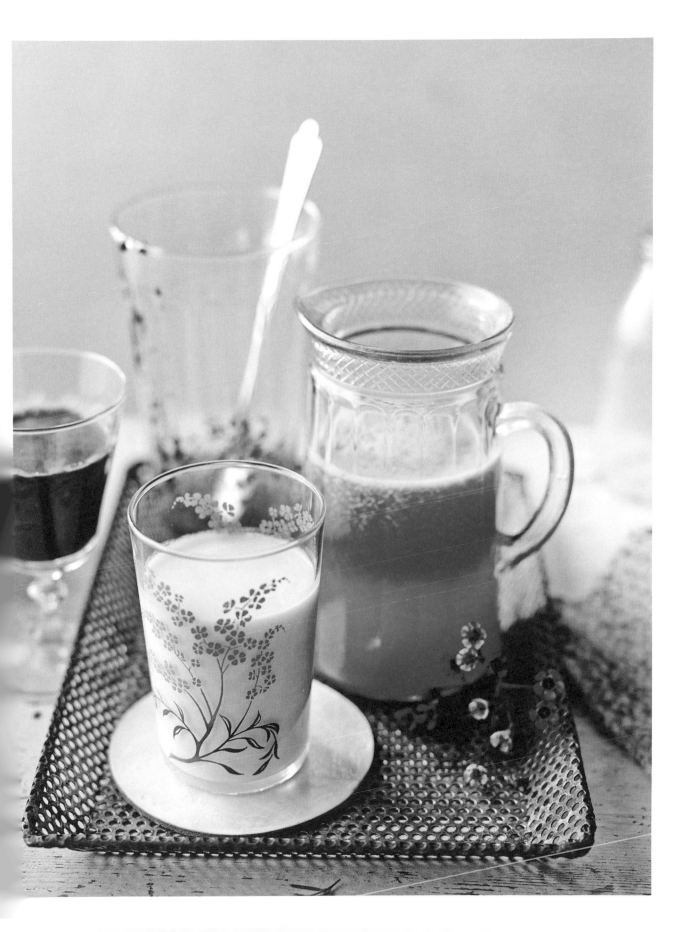

skin

These skin-loving drinks will pump you full of goodness, making your skin glow ever brighter. All serve one person.

drink your five-a-day

1 handful kale
2 carrots
1 apple, peeled and cored
1 pear, peeled and cored
1 lemon, peeled and pith removed

Put all the ingredients into a juicer. Drink that day.

skin saver

7 sticks celery
1 apple, peeled and cored
½ cucumber
1 handful parsley
1 handful spinach leaves
juice of 1 lemon
juice of 1 lime

Put all the ingredients into a juicer. Drink that day.

almond milk

Most shop-bought almond milks are packed with nasty chemicals and added sugar. Making your own ... well, it's super simple. Just soak, blend and sip.

100g almonds
300ml water
1 tsp cinnamon
pinch salt

Soak the almonds in enough water to cover for 6–12 hours.

Discard the almond soaking water, and rinse the almonds in a sieve under running water.

Put the soaked almonds, 300ml water, the cinnamon and salt in a blender. Blend for 4 minutes, then strain through a nut milk bag or piece of muslin. Squeeze the cloth to extract excess liquid.

The milk will keep for a week in a container in the fridge.

beauty juice

3 sticks celery
2 handfuls spinach
2 pears, peeled and cored
1 cucumber
1 lemon, peeled and pith removed
1 handful parsley

Put all the ingredients into a juicer. Drink that day.

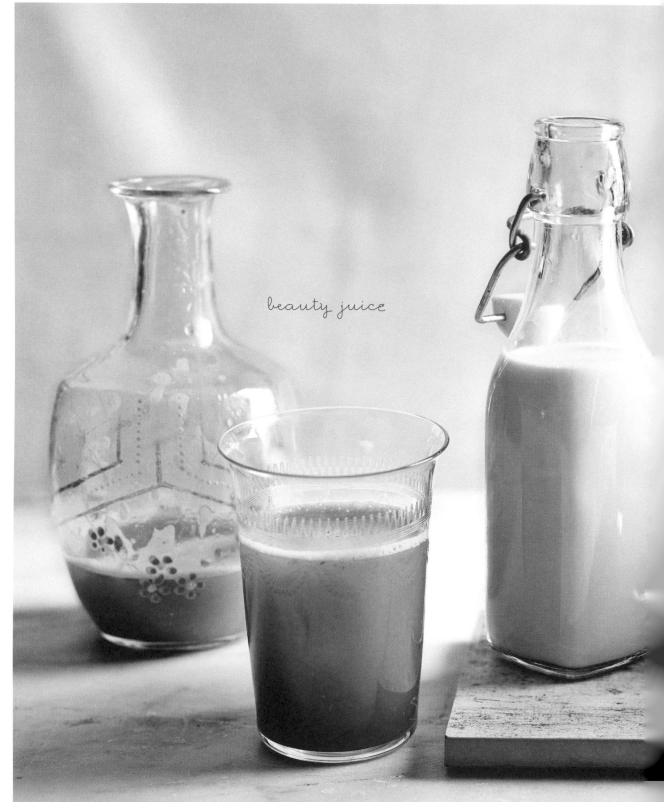

beauty juice

almond milk

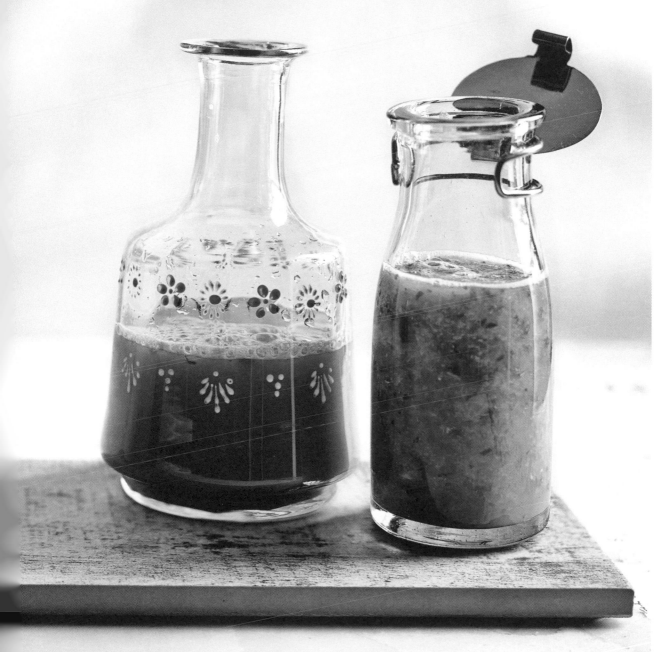

skin saver

drink your five-a-day

de-stress

Wind down with these nourishing drinks, all designed to relax, restore and repair the body. All serve one person.

date and cardamom almond milk

This gorgeous warm milk is spiced with the flavours of India – perfect as a nightcap. The cinnamon gives it a nice sweetness and helps to regulate your blood sugar levels and reduce later cravings.

300ml almond milk
1 whole cardamom pod
5 Medjool dates, stones removed
1 cinnamon stick

Blend the milk with the cardamom and dates for 2 minutes, then strain through a fine sieve.

Pour the milk into a saucepan and heat to a low simmer with the cinnamon stick for 5 minutes. Pour into mugs to enjoy.

stir and purr (sleep tonic)

1 green apple, peeled and cored
7 strawberries, hulled
15 cherries, stones removed
2 sticks celery
½ cucumber

Put all the ingredients into a juicer. Drink that day.

hangover helper

3 medium tomatoes
1 stick celery
1 lemon
2.5cm piece ginger, peeled
1 jalapeño chilli, seeds removed
½ cucumber

Put all the ingredients into a juicer. Drink that day.

hot chocolate

This is like a hug in a mug, spiced with cinnamon
as well as cacao. Enjoy this one with giant socks and
a big rug.

250ml almond or coconut milk
1 tbsp raw cacao
1 tsp cinnamon
1 tsp coconut sugar

Warm the milk, cacao, cinnamon and coconut sugar in a saucepan
over a low to medium heat. Pour into mugs to enjoy.

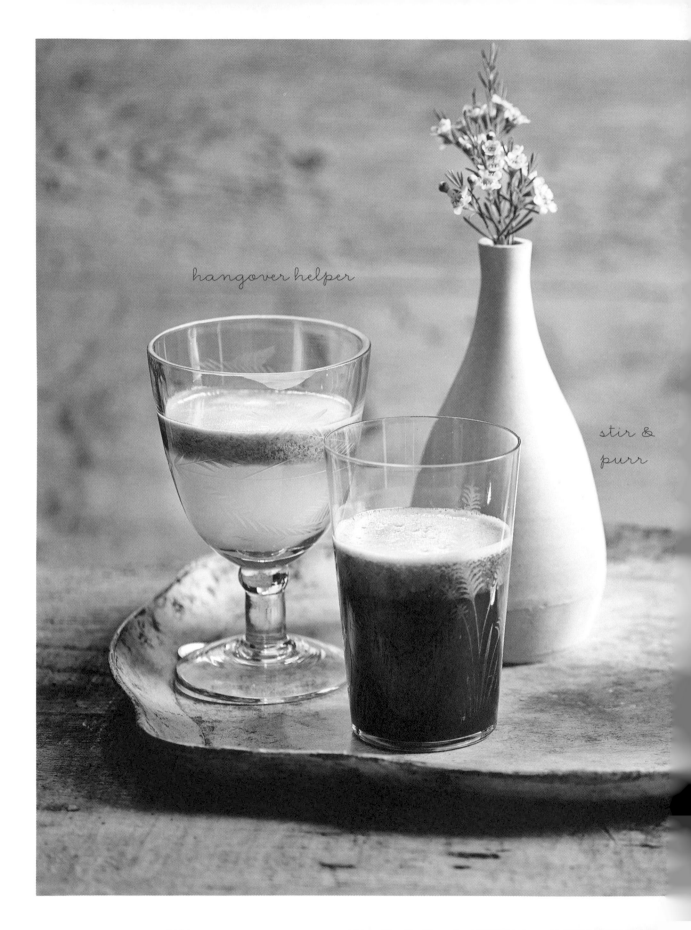

hangover helper

stir &
purr

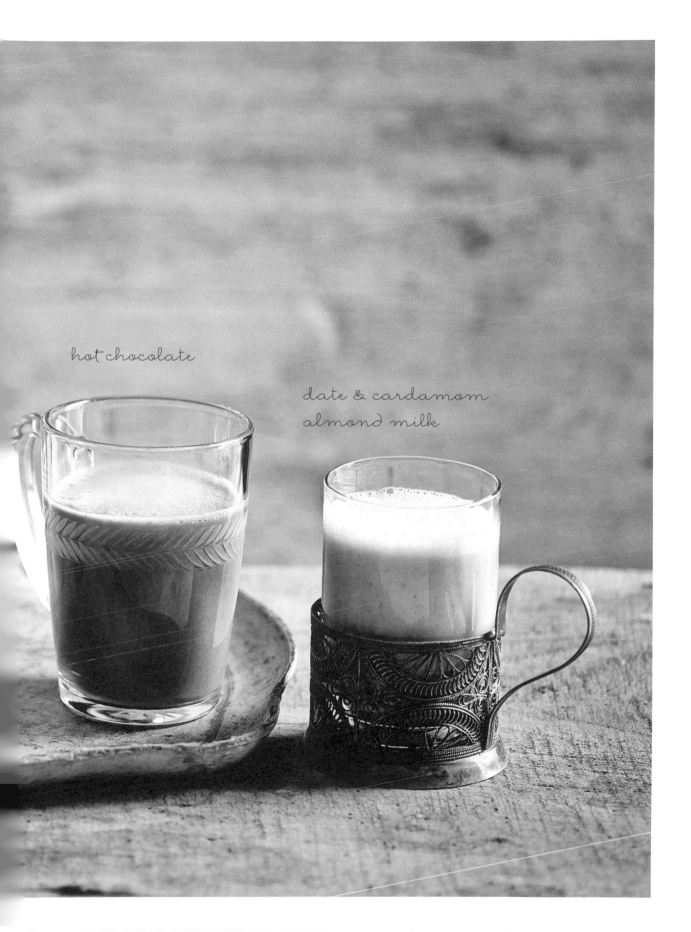

hot chocolate

date & cardamom
almond milk

index

acknowledgements

Thank you to my amazing boyfriend Kieran for making me smile everyday. To my gorgeous manager Alice for believing in me and making this dream come true. To all the amazing people who made this book the beauty it is. To my family, my biggest cheerleaders, thank you for helping me chase my dreams. Finally a big thank you to you, for buying this book, and spreading the *Get the Glow* philosophy. Let's enjoy this journey together.

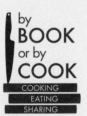

by
BOOK
or by
COOK
COOKING
EATING
SHARING

For lots more delicious recipes plus articles, interviews and videos from the best chefs cooking today visit our blog
bybookorbycook.co.uk

Follow us
 @bybookorbycook

Find us
 facebook.com/bybookorbycook

Copyright © Madeleine Shaw 2015

The right of Madeleine Shaw to be identified as the author of this work has been asserted in accordance with the Copyright, Designs and Patents Act 1988.

This edition first published in Great Britain in 2015 by Orion, an imprint of the Orion Publishing Group Ltd,
Orion House, 5 Upper St Martin's Lane,
London WC2H 9EA
An Hachette UK Company

10 9 8 7

A CIP catalogue record for this book is available from the British Library.

ISBN: 978-1-4091-5744-1

Photography: Martin Poole, Ellis Parrinder
Design: Arielle Gamble
Food styling: Bianca Nice
Prop styling: Olivia Wardle

Food photography © Martin Poole with the exception of the following: Holly Clark: page 22 (bottom left), 32 (top left/ bottom right), 50 (top left/ bottom right); Tommy Clarke: page 27 (top right); Josh Kearns: page 12 (right), 37 (all except bottom left), 63, 68 (top right), 100 (bottom left), 214 (bottom left); Ellis Parrinder: page 4 (top right), 10, 20, 30, 38, 48, 56, 114 (bottom right), 154 (bottom right), 186 (top left), 253 (bottom); Madeleine Shaw: page 50 (bottom left).

Printed in Italy

The Orion Publishing Group's policy is to use papers that are natural, renewable and recyclable and made from wood grown in sustainable forests. The logging and manufacturing processes are expected to conform to the environmental regulations of the country of origin.

Every effort has been made to fulfil requirements with regard to reproducing copyright material. The author and publisher will be glad to rectify any omissions at the earliest opportunity.

www.orionbooks.co.uk